CONTENTS

3

4

INTRODUCTION

For many people, fried food is the absolute comfort food. Whether it's fried chicken, French fries, or fried street food, everyone has probably at least one fried food included on their guilt list.

Having tried it yourself, you know that frying makes your food taste delicious and crispy. However, while the flavor of foods burst in your mouth, sometimes you just can't help but think about how much calories you get from eating greasy foods.

Well, that's right, we all know how it's done. You need oil to fry, oftentimes, you need lots of it. And from what we know, too much oil on food is bad news. But did you know that it is actually possible to have tasty and crunchy food without having to drench your meal in oil?

Air fryers have become some of the hottest kitchen appliances today that make frying easier without the guilt. This kitchen gadget was invented to replace your traditional oil fryer with air to make it a healthy alternative to frying with oil. This new innovation has been gaining footing in many countries in the west and thus far has been making a difference in the way households prepare their food.

By definition, an air fryer is a kitchen appliance that cooks food by circulating hot air via convection mechanism. The hot air is circulated at high speed around the food by a mechanical fan, cooking the food and making it crispy.

In America, the grave effects of obesity have been associated with the consumption of too much oily food. The use of air fryers has been gaining praises due to its promising offer as a healthy solution to the long existing problem of obesity as a result of eating oil-filled food. Its auspicious contribution in the making a healthier lifestyle through healthy eating is what makes these types of gizmos very appealing especially to those who are trying to lose weight and those who are aiming for healthier living.

For those who can't live without fried food, using an air fryer is a good choice to cut down fat and calories from your food. Less oil means fewer calories.

Essentials of Ninja Air Fryer Max XL

Do you ever find yourself short on time to cook? Perhaps, trying to cut down your weight but can't let go of those fatty food? Are you looking for a great kitchen tool to invest that can make any meal prep easier without much hassle?

When it comes to modern day cooking, one of the coolest gadgets that you can own in your household is an air fryer that does it all—a real ninja in the kitchen.

Ninja is one big name in the kitchen gadget scene. While it is best known for its blenders, this company is one of the best makers of the best air fryers in the market. With its sleek black design and high functionality of its air fryers, every unit looks great in any kitchen.

If you have been contemplating on whether an air fryer is worth the purchase, you may want to know what it does for you. At fingertips, you can have an appliance that can imitate foods made in oil fryers, only that it is healthier and guilt-free with Ninja Air Fryer Max XL. This air fryer will serves up many ways in making life easier. Definitely a wise choice for every household.

What is Ninja Air Fryer Max XL?

Ninja Air Fryer Max XL (Ninja AF161 Series) offers a fast and easy way of preparing your favorite food.

This Ninja fryer can cook your favorite food to crisp using little to no oil, making food preparation healthier.

Skip the take-out and prepare tasty and healthy fried meals minus the guilt in a flash. This appliance fries up with 75% less fat than any other frying methods. Less oils, less calories.

How the Ninja Air Fryer Max XL Works?

Ninja Air Fryer Max XL uses Max Crisp Technology that cooks food for up to 30 percent faster than the Ninja AF100 Series.

It has a family-sized 5.5-qt basket can cook up to 3-lb French fries, chicken tenders and more and make them crunchy and chewy in no time minus the grease.

Aside from air frying, its other functions include **Max Crisp, Air Roast, Air Broil, Bake, Reheat and Dehydrate.**

Make healthy meals in a flash with this Ninja Air Fryer series.

Is Ninja Air Fryer Max XL Better Than Normal Air Fryer?

Most air fryers replace traditional deep fryers due to its promising benefits as far as food quality and convenience are concerned. However, not all air fryers offer the same quality, so it is important to choose the right product for you to get the best out of this great kitchen innovation. Since the invention of this genius gadget, there are now a lot of air fryers that exist in the market claiming to be the best appliance that suit your cooking needs so it all boils down to quality.

Ninja Air Fryer Max XL works like a real ninja. It cooks your food perfectly and fast plus it's easy to use by anyone in the household. This unit offers a simple set of push-button controls of its functions that works immediately at one press of your fingertips. It has various cooking functions that easily activates with a push of the button. Select from max crisp, air fry, air roast, air broil, bake, reheat, and dehydrate.

The Ninja Air Fryers Series has multi-function features. The number of functions varies between air fryer models. The Ninja Air Fryer Max XL is bigger in dimension so it fits a lot of food that you can cook at once.

Ninja Air Fryer Max XL delivers 110 degrees to 450 degrees of superheated air that turns food into a scrumptious meal.

It works by circulating hot air around the food using the convection mechanism. A built-in mechanical fan circulates the hot air around the food at high speed, cooking the food and producing a crispy layer via browning reactions.

This ninja air fryer allows food to be cooked on its own oil and releasing them which lessens the oil content for a guilt-free fried meal favorites.

Buttons and Functions

The Ninja Air Fryer Max XL offers button controls that are easy to use so that anyone can operate it.

Cooking Functions Buttons

Max Crisp

Select this function to give frozen foods extra crispiness and crunch with little to no oil.

Air Fry

Use this function to give food crispiness and crunch with little to no oil.

Air Roast

This can be used to roast tender meats, vegetables, and more.

Air Broil

Use this function to caramelize and brown food.

Bake

Select this function to create decedent baked treats and desserts such as tarts and cookies.

Reheat

Functions similar to a microwave that heats leftovers by gently warming them, leaving you with crispy, fresh tasting heated food.

Dehydrate

Use this function to dehydrate meats, fruits, and vegetables for healthy snacks.

Operating Buttons

The Ninja Air Fryer Max XL has operating buttons that are easy to use in setting up functions and cooking settings.

Temp Arrows

Adjust the cooking temperature for any function by pressing the UP and DOWN buttons before or during cooking. Preheat the fryer by setting the temperature using these buttons.

Time Arrows

Adjust the cooking time for any function using the UP and DOWN buttons.

Start/Stop Button

After setting the time and temperature, press START/STOP button to start cooking. Press the same button to stop cooking.

Power Button

Turn ON/OFF the unit by pressing the Power button. This also stops all cooking modes of the fryer.

How to Use it Properly

Before Using Ninja Air Fryer Max XL

Ninja Air Fryer Max XL is strategically designed to provide convenience in cooking. Its unit design and features are easy to operate for a no mess no stress food preparation.

● Remove and discard all the unnecessary packaging material from the unit. Remove all accessories from the package.

● Read the user's manual carefully. Pay close attention to operational instructions, warnings, and important safeguards to safely use the unit and avoid accidents.

● Wash the ceramic-coated basket, crisper plate, and accessories in hot, soapy water, then rinse and dry thoroughly before using. NEVER clean the main unit in the dishwasher.

Using the Cooking Functions

Plug the power cord into a wall outlet and press the Power button to turn on the unit.

Max Crisp

1.   Attach the crisper plate in the basket.
2.   Press the MAX CRISP button. The default temperature setting will be displayed on the screen. (The temperature setup CANNOT be changed in this function.)
3.   Set the cooking time by pressing the TIME buttons.
4.   Add the ingredients to be cooked to the basket. Insert the basket in the unit.
5.   Press START/STOP button to start cooking.
6.   Remove the basket and toss the ingredients. (The unit will pause cooking automatically when the basket is removed and will resume once the basket is reinserted.)
7.   The unit will beep and END will display on the control panel when cooking is complete.
8.   Remove the ingredients from the basket.
Note: For best results, preheat the fryer for 3 minutes before adding the ingredients.

Air Fry

1.   Attach the crisper plate in the basket.
2.   Press the AIR FRY button. The default temperature setting will be displayed on the screen. Set the desired frying temperature using the TEMP buttons.
3.   Set the frying time by pressing the TIME buttons.
4.   Add the ingredients to be cooked to the basket. Insert the basket in the unit.
5.   Press START/STOP button to start cooking.
6.   Remove the basket and toss the ingredients. (The unit will pause cooking automatically when the basket is removed and will resume once the basket is reinserted.)
7.   The unit will beep and END will display on the control panel when frying is complete.
8.   Remove the ingredients from the basket.
Note: For best results, preheat the fryer for 3 minutes before adding the ingredients.

Air Roast

1.   Attach the crisper plate in the basket.
2.   Press the AIR ROAST button. The default temperature setting will be displayed on the screen. Set the desired roasting temperature using the TEMP buttons.
3.   Set the roasting time by pressing the TIME buttons.
4.   Add the ingredients to be cooked to the basket. Insert the basket in the unit.
5.   Press START/STOP button to start cooking.
6.   Remove the basket and toss the ingredients. (The unit will pause cooking automatically when the basket is removed and will resume once the basket is reinserted.)
7.   The unit will beep and END will display on the control panel when roasting is complete.
8.   Remove the ingredients from the basket.
Note: For best results, preheat the fryer for 3 minutes before adding the ingredients.

Air Broil

1.   Attach the crisper plate in the basket.

2. Press the AIR BROIL button. The default temperature setting will be displayed on the screen. Set the desired broiling temperature using the TEMP buttons.

3. Set the broiling time by pressing the TIME buttons.

4. Add the ingredients to be cooked to the basket. Insert the basket in the unit. Recommended: Preheat heater for 3 minutes before adding ingredients

5. Press START/STOP button to start cooking.

6. Remove the basket and toss the ingredients. (The unit will pause cooking automatically when the basket is removed and will resume once the basket is reinserted.)

7. The unit will beep and END will display on the control panel when broiling is complete.

8. Remove the ingredients from the basket.

Note: For best results, use the broil rack. When using the broil rack, do not layer food below the rack.

Bake

1. Attach the crisper plate in the basket.

2. Press the BAKE button. The default temperature setting will be displayed on the screen. Set the desired baking temperature using the TEMP buttons.

3. Set the baking time by pressing the TIME buttons.

4. Add the ingredients to be cooked to the basket. Insert the basket in the unit. Recommended: Preheat heater for 3 minutes before adding ingredients

5. Press START/STOP button to start cooking.

6. The unit will beep and END will display on the control panel when baking is complete.

7. Remove the ingredients from the basket.

Note: To convert recipes from a conventional oven, reduce the temperature of the air fryer by 25°F. Check food frequently to avoid overcooking.

Reheat

1. Attach the crisper plate in the basket.

2. Press the REHEAT button. The default temperature setting will be displayed on the screen. Set the desired reheating temperature using the TEMP buttons.

3. Set there heating time by pressing the TIME buttons.

4. Add the ingredients to be cooked to the basket. Insert the basket in the unit. Press START/STOP button to start cooking.

5. The unit will beep and END will display on the control panel when reheating is complete.

6. Remove the ingredients from the basket.

Dehydrate

1. Arrange the layer of ingredients in the bottom of the basket then install the crisper plate for a set of second layer of ingredients.

2. Press the DEHYDRATE button. The default temperature setting will be displayed on the screen. Set the desired dehydrating temperature using the TEMP buttons.

3. Set the dehydrating time by pressing the TIME buttons.

4.   Add the ingredients to be cooked to the basket. Insert the basket in the unit. Press START/STOP button to start cooking.

5.   The unit will beep and END will display on the control panel when dehydrating is complete.

6.   Remove the ingredients from the basket.

Note: You can increase your air fryer's dehydrating capacity with the mid-level rack.

Where to Shop For it

The Ninja Air Fryer Max XL can be purchased at Amazon at a retail price of $139.99. This Ninja Air Fryer is rated 4.7 out of 5 stars in Amazon.

Safety Guide on Using it

Here is a guide on how to safely use the Ninja Air Fryer Max XL:

• Read the user's manual to know how to operate the unit.

• Always ensure that all the parts of the appliance are properly assembled before use.

• Make sure that the air intake vent or air socket vent are not blocked while the unit is running. Doing so may cause overheat to the unit or may facilitate uneven cooking.

• Ensure that the removable ceramic coated basket is clean and dry before placing it into the main unit.

• The Ninja Air Fryer Max XL is made for household use only. Do not use outdoors.

• This unit is intended for worktop use only. Ensure that the surface is clean, dry and leveled. Do not move the unit when in use.

• Do not touch hot surface. Always wear protective hot pads or oven mitts when using the appliance to prevent burns or personal injury.

• Do not place the appliance near hot surfaces and flammables such as hot gas or electric burner.

• If the unit emits black smoke, unplug the unit immediately and wait for the smoking to stop before taking out the other accessories.

How to Clean Your Air Fryer Max XL

Always ensure that the accessories are clean and dry before and after every use.

• Unplug the unit prior to cleaning. Never immerse the main unit in water or any other liquid or place in a dishwasher.

• Clean the main unit and the control panel with a damp cloth. While the basket, crisper plate and other accessories can be washed with water or can be cleaned in the dishwasher.

• If food is stuck on the crisper plate or basket, allow it to smoke in warm soapy water to soften the residues.

• Air- dry or towel-dry all parts after cleaning.

Amazing Tips and Tricks on Using it

1. Do not overcrowd the ingredients.

To facilitate even cooking and browning, make sure the ingredients are properly arranged and do not overlap in the basket. Check the food and shake the basket for even browning.

2. Convert oven recipes.

Convert oven recipes by reducing the temperature of the fryer by 25°F. check thecheck progress frequently to avoid overcooking. Remove food when desired level of brownness has been achieved.

3. Preheat

Preheat the fryer for 3 minutes before placing the ingredients to ensure even temperature inside the unit.

4. Secure your food.

Secure lightweight foods with toothpicks inside the fryer as they may be blown inside by the mechanical fan.

5. Add more crisp.

Use the crisper plate to improve crispiness of the ingredients. The crisper plate will lift the ingredients in the basket so air can circulate all over the food for a more crisp result.

6. Add a bit of oil.

When cooking fresh vegetables, use at least 1 tablespoon of oil and add more to achieve a preferred level of crispine.

Dehydrate Tips & Tricks

1. Make thin slices.

Make thin slices to achieve perfectly dehydrated food slices. To make consistent thin slices, use a mandoline slice to get thin fruits and vegetable slices.

2. Dry your ingredients.

Pat the ingredients dry before placing them in the basket to remove excess moisture or liquids.

3. Trim off the fat.

Fat does not dry out and may turn rancid. Trim off the fat of the beef or poultry before dehydrating them.

4. Do not overcrowd.

Lay the ingredients flat on the basket, closely as possible but not overlapping. Optimize the space to avoid uneven drying of the ingredients.

5. Use Roast Function to pasteurize jerky.

When dehydrating meats, finish it off by using the Roast function at 330°F for 1 minute to fully pasteurize the dried meat.

6. Store the dried ingredients well.

Store the dehydrated foods at room temperature in an airtight container for up to 2 weeks to maximize its shelf lie.

FAQS

1. How high can the temperature of the fryer go?

For Max Crisp and Air boil, the temperature can go at a maximum of 450 degrees F while the max temperature for all function is 400 degrees F.

2. How long do I need to preheat the air fryer? How will I know when it's done?

To preheat, select the function, time and temperature of the air fryer, and press START/STOP. We recommend preheating the fryer for 3 minutes.

3. What are the cooking functions included in the unit?

The air fryer unit has 7 different cooking functions: Max Crisp, Air Broil, Air Fry, Dehydrate, Air Roast, Bake, and Reheat (Max Crisp and Air Broil not included in all models).

4. Should you defrost the frozen foods before air frying?

This depends on the kind of food you are going to fry. For frozen meats, it's better to defrost them first prior to air drying.

5. When should I add the ingredients? Can I put the item before or after preheating?

Allow the unit to preheat first for at least 3 minutes prior to adding the ingredients to get best result.

6. How do I pause the countdown?

Removing the basket from the unit will automatically pause the timer. If you want to totally stop the cooking function, press START/STOP to reset the timer.

7. Is the basket non-stick? When do I use the crisper plate?

The basket is made from aluminum with a non-stick ceramic coating. The crisper plate raises the food in the basket to allow air to flow under it as it cooks, this way your food is cooked evenly and turns out crispy.

8. My food didn't cook well. Why?

The cook time and temperature can be adjusted at any time. Check your food a few times while it cooks. Simply press the TIME or TEMP buttons and rotate the dial. Make sure to arrange the ingredients in the basket in an even layer. Do not overlap the ingredients so it will brown evenly on all sides. Always make sure that the basket is fully inserted as it cooks.

9. Why did my food burn?

To avoid overcooking, check progress throughout cooking to see how your food is. Remove the food from the basket once you get your desired outcome.

10. Can I air fry fresh battered foods?

Yes, but the ingredients need to be breaded properly. It needs to be coated flour, egg and crumbs in a way that it sticks properly in place unto the food pieces. Loose breading may be blown off by the fryer's fan. The food must not be wetly coated with the batter as well as it will only run down and will stick to the basket instead as it fries.

11. Why do some ingredients get blown when air frying?

The fryer has a fan inside which may blow lightweight foods around. You can use

12. The screen suddenly went black. What happened?

If the screen turns black when you didn't turn it off means it went on standby mode. Press the power button to turn it back on.

13. What does the beeping of the unit means?

When the timer sets off, the unit will start beeping indicating the cooking function is complete.

14. What does an "E" on the display screen means?

This indicates ERROR and the unit may not be functioning properly.

BREAKFAST & BRUNCH RECIPES

1. Shrimp Stuff Peppers

Servings: 6
Cooking Time: 6 Minutes
Ingredients:
- 12 baby bell peppers, cut into halves
- 1 tbsp olive oil
- 1 tbsp fresh lemon juice
- ¼ cup basil pesto
- 1 lb shrimp, cooked
- ½ tsp red pepper flakes, crushed
- 2 tbsp parsley, chopped
- Pepper
- Salt

Directions:
1. In a bowl, mix together shrimp, parsley, red pepper flakes, basil pesto, lemon juice, oil, pepper, and salt.
2. Stuff shrimp mixture into the bell pepper halved and place into the air fryer basket.
3. Cook at 320 F for 6 minutes.
4. Serve and enjoy.

2. Potato Rosti

Servings:2
Cooking Time: 15 Minutes
Ingredients:
- 1 teaspoon olive oil
- ½ pound russet potatoes, peeled and roughly grated
- 1 tablespoon fresh chives, finely chopped
- Salt and ground black pepper, as required
- 2 tablespoons sour cream
- 3½ ounces smoked salmon, cut into slices

Directions:
1. Set the temperature of Air Fryer to 355 degrees F. Grease a pizza pan with the olive oil.
2. In a large bowl, mix together the potatoes, chives, salt, and black pepper.
3. Place the potato mixture into the prepared pizza pan.
4. Arrange the pan in an Air Fryer basket.
5. Air Fry for about 15 minutes or until the top becomes golden brown.
6. Cut the potato rosti into wedges.
7. Top with the sour cream and smoked salmon slices and serve immediately.

3. Dill Egg Rolls

Servings: 4
Cooking Time: 4 Minutes
Ingredients:
- 2 eggs, hard-boiled, peeled
- 1 tablespoon cream cheese
- 1 tablespoon fresh dill, chopped
- 1 teaspoon ground black pepper
- 4 wontons wrap
- 1 egg white, whisked
- 1 teaspoon sesame oil

Directions:
1. Chop the eggs and mix them up with cream cheese, dill, and ground black pepper. Then place the egg mixture on the wonton wraps and roll them into the rolls. Brush every roll with whisked egg white. After this, preheat the air fryer to 395F and brush the air fryer basket with sesame oil. Arrange the egg rolls in the hot air fryer and cook them for 2 minutes from each side or until the rolls are golden brown.

4. The Simplest Grilled Cheese

Servings:1
Cooking Time: 10 Minutes
Ingredients:
- 2 slices bread
- 3 slices American cheese

Directions:
1. Preheat the air fryer to 370 F. Spread one tsp of butter on the outside of each of the bread slices. Place the cheese on the inside of one bread slice. Top with the other slice. Cook in the air fryer for 4 minutes. Flip the sandwich over and cook for an additional 4 minutes. Serve cut diagonally.

5. Lemony Raspberries

Servings: 2
Cooking Time: 12 Minutes
Ingredients:
- 1 cup raspberries
- 2 tablespoons lemon juice
- 2 tablespoons butter
- 1 teaspoon cinnamon powder

Directions:
1. In your air fryer, mix all the ingredients, toss, cover, cook at 350 degrees F for 12 minutes, divide into bowls and serve for breakfast.

6. Toasted Cheese

Servings: 2
Cooking Time: 20 Minutes
Ingredients:
- 2 slices bread
- 4 oz cheese, grated
- Small amount of butter

Directions:
1. Grill the bread in the toaster.
2. Butter the toast and top with the grated cheese.
3. Set your Air Fryer to 350°F and allow to warm.

4. Put the toast slices inside the fryer and cook for 4 - 6 minutes.
5. Serve and enjoy!

7. Bok Choy And Egg Frittata

Servings:2
Cooking Time:8 Minutes
Ingredients:
- 1 cup bok choy, chopped
- 2 eggs
- 2 tablespoons milk
- 1 tablespoon cheddar cheese, grated
- 1 tablespoon feta cheese, grated
- Salt and black pepper, to taste
- 1 tablespoon olive oil

Directions:
1. Preheat the Air fryer to 360 °F and grease an Air Fryer pan.
2. Whisk together eggs with milk, salt and black pepper in a bowl.
3. Heat olive oil in the Air Fryer pan and add bok choy.
4. Cook for about 3 minutes and stir in the whisked eggs.
5. Top with cheese and cook for about 5 minutes.
6. Dish out and serve hot.

8. Egg Muffins

Servings: 1
Cooking Time: 30 Minutes
Ingredients:
- 1 tbsp green pesto
- oz/75g shredded cheese
- oz/150g cooked bacon
- 1 scallion, chopped
- eggs

Directions:
1. You should set your fryer to 350°F/175°C.
2. Place liners in a regular cupcake tin. This will help with easy removal and storage.
3. Beat the eggs with pepper, salt, and the pesto. Mix in the cheese.
4. Pour the eggs into the cupcake tin and top with the bacon and scallion.
5. Cook for 15-20 minutes, or until the egg is set.

9. English Egg Breakfast

Servings: 2
Cooking Time: 25 Minutes
Ingredients:
- 2 cups flour
- 1 cup pumpkin puree
- 1 tbsp. oil
- 2 tbsp. vinegar
- 2 tsp baking powder
- ½ cup milk
- 2 eggs

- 1 tsp. baking soda
- 1 tbsp. sugar
- 1 tsp. cinnamon powder

Directions:
1. Set your Air Fryer at 300°F to pre-heat.
2. Crack the eggs into a bowl and beat with a whisk. Combine with the milk, flour, baking powder, sugar, pumpkin purée, cinnamon powder, and baking soda, mixing well and adding more milk if necessary.
3. Grease the baking tray with oil. Add in the mixture and transfer into the Air Fryer. Cook for 10 minutes.

10. Spiced Cauliflower And Ham Quiche

Servings: 4
Cooking Time: 15 Minutes
Ingredients:
- 5 eggs, beaten
- ½ cup heavy cream
- 1 teaspoon ground nutmeg
- ¼ teaspoon ground cardamom
- ¼ teaspoon salt
- 1 teaspoon ground black pepper
- 1 teaspoon butter, softened
- ¼ cup spring onions, chopped
- ¼ cup cauliflower florets
- 5 oz ham, chopped
- 3 oz Provolone cheese, grated

Directions:
1. Pour the beaten eggs in the bowl. Add heavy cream, ground nutmeg, ground cardamom, ground black pepper, and salt. After this, pour the liquid in the air fryer round pan. Add butter, onion, cauliflower florets, ham, and cheese. Gently stir the quiche liquid. Place it in the air fryer and cook the quiche for 15 minutes at 385F.

11. Sweet Potato Hash

Servings:6
Cooking Time:15 Minutes
Ingredients:
- 2 large sweet potato, cut into small cubes
- 2 slices bacon, cut into small pieces
- 2 tablespoons olive oil
- 1 tablespoon smoked paprika
- 1 teaspoon sea salt
- 1 teaspoon ground black pepper
- 1 teaspoon dried dill weed

Directions:
1. Preheat the Air Fryer to 400 °F and grease an Air fryer pan.
2. Mix together sweet potato, bacon, olive oil, paprika, salt, black pepper and dill in a large bowl.
3. Transfer the mixture into the preheated air fryer pan and cook for about 15 minutes, stirring in between.

4. Dish out and serve warm.

12. Hash Brown

Servings: 2
Cooking Time: 20 Minutes
Ingredients:
- 12 oz grated fresh cauliflower (about ½ a medium-sized head)
- 4 slices bacon, chopped
- 3 oz onion, chopped
- 1 tbsp butter, softened

Directions:
1. In a skillet, sauté the bacon and onion until brown.
2. Add in the cauliflower and stir until tender and browned.
3. Add the butter steadily as it cooks.
4. Season to taste with salt and pepper.
5. Enjoy!

13. Protein-rich Breakfast

Servings: 4
Cooking Time: 23 Minutes
Ingredients:
- 1 tablespoon unsalted butter, melted
- 1 pound fresh baby spinach
- 4 eggs
- 7-ounces ham, sliced
- 4 teaspoons milk
- 1 tablespoon olive oil
- Salt and black pepper, to taste

Directions:
1. Preheat the Air fryer to 355 °F and grease 4 ramekins with butter.
2. Heat olive oil on medium heat in a skillet and add spinach.
3. Cook for about 3 minutes until wilted and drain the liquid completely from the spinach.
4. Divide the spinach into prepared ramekins and top with ham slices.
5. Crack 1 egg over ham slices into each ramekin and drizzle with milk evenly.
6. Season with salt and black pepper and transfer into the Air fryer.
7. Bake for about 20 minutes and serve hot.

14. Greek Vegetables

Servings: 6
Cooking Time: 35 Minutes
Ingredients:
- 1 eggplant, sliced
- 4 tomatoes, quarters
- 2 onion, chopped
- 1 thyme sprig, chopped
- 1 bay leaf
- 3 tbsp olive oil
- 3 garlic cloves, minced
- 2 bell peppers, chopped
- 1 zucchini, sliced
- Pepper
- Salt

Directions:
1. Add all ingredients into the air fryer baking pan and mix well.
2. Place pan in the air fryer and cook at 300 F for 35 minutes.
3. Serve and enjoy.

15. American Donuts

Servings: 6
Cooking Time: 1 Hour 20 Minutes
Ingredients:
- 1 cup flour
- ¼ cup sugar
- 1 tsp. baking powder
- ½ tsp. salt
- ¼ tsp. cinnamon
- 1 tbsp. coconut oil, melted
- 2 tbsp. aquafaba or liquid from canned chickpeas
- ¼ cup milk

Directions:
1. Put the sugar, flour and baking powder in a bowl and combine. Mix in the salt and cinnamon.
2. In a separate bowl, combine the aquafaba, milk and coconut oil.
3. Slowly pour the dry ingredients into the wet ingredients and combine well to create a sticky dough.
4. Refrigerate for at least an hour.
5. Pre-heat your Air Fryer at 370°F.
6. Using your hands, shape the dough into several small balls and place each one inside the fryer. Cook for 10 minutes, refraining from shaking the basket as they cook.
7. Lightly dust the balls with sugar and cinnamon and serve with a hot cup of coffee.

16. Bacon Egg Muffins

Servings: 12
Cooking Time: 20 Minutes
Ingredients:
- 12 eggs
- 2 tbsp fresh parsley, chopped
- 1/2 tsp mustard powder
- 1/3 cup heavy cream
- 2 green onion, chopped
- 4 oz cheddar cheese, shredded
- 8 bacon slices, cooked and crumbled
- Pepper
- Salt

Directions:
1. Preheat the air fryer to 350 F.

2. In a mixing bowl, whisk together eggs, mustard powder, heavy cream, pepper, and salt.
3. Divide cheddar cheese, onions, and bacon into the silicone muffin molds.
4. Now pour egg mixture into the silicone muffin molds and place in the air fryer basket.
5. Cook muffins for 20 minutes.
6. Serve and enjoy.

17. Cheesy Omelet

Servings:1
Cooking Time: 15 Minutes
Ingredients:
- Black pepper to taste
- 1 cup cheddar cheese, shredded
- 1 whole onion, chopped
- 2 tbsp soy sauce

Directions:
1. Preheat your air fryer to 340 F. Drizzle soy sauce over the chopped onions. Place the onions in your air fryer's cooking basket and cook for 8 minutes. In a bowl, mix the beaten eggs with salt and pepper.
2. Pour the egg mixture over onions (in the cooking basket) and cook for 3 minutes. Add cheddar cheese over eggs and bake for 2 more minutes. Serve with fresh basil and enjoy!

18. Basil Tomato Bowls

Servings: 4
Cooking Time: 15 Minutes
Ingredients:
- 1 pound cherry tomatoes, halved
- 1 cup mozzarella, shredded
- Cooking spray
- Salt and black pepper to the taste
- 1 teaspoon basil, chopped

Directions:
1. Grease the tomatoes with the cooking spray, season with salt and pepper, sprinkle the mozzarella on top, place them all in your air fryer's basket, cook at 330 degrees F for 15 minutes, divide into bowls, sprinkle the basil on top and serve.

19. Bread & Bacon Cups

Servings:2
Cooking Time: 10 Minutes
Ingredients:
- ½ teaspoon butter
- 2 bread slices
- 1 bacon slice, chopped
- 4 tomato slices
- 1 tablespoon Mozzarella cheese, shredded
- 2 eggs
- 1/8 teaspoon maple syrup

- 1/8 teaspoon balsamic vinegar
- ¼ teaspoon fresh parsley, chopped
- Salt and freshly ground pepper, to taste
- 2 tablespoons mayonnaise

Directions:
1. Set the temperature of Air Fryer to 320 degrees F. Lightly, grease 2 ramekins.
2. Line each prepared ramekin with 1 bread slice.
3. Divide evenly the bacon and tomato slices over bread slice in each ramekin.
4. Top evenly with the cheese.
5. Crack 1 egg in each ramekin over cheese.
6. Drizzle with maple syrup and vinegar and then sprinkle with parsley, salt and black pepper.
7. Place the ramekins in an Air Fryer basket.
8. Air Fry for 10 minutes or until desired doneness.
9. Top with mayonnaise and serve.

20. Blueberry Muffins

Servings:12
Cooking Time: 12 Minutes
Ingredients:
- 2 cups plus 2 tablespoons self-rising flour
- 5 tablespoons white sugar
- ½ cup milk
- 2 ounces butter, melted
- 2 eggs
- 2 teaspoons fresh orange zest, finely grated
- 2 tablespoons fresh orange juice
- ½ teaspoon vanilla extract
- ½ cup fresh blueberries

Directions:
1. In a bowl, mix together the flour, and white sugar.
2. In another large bowl, mix well the remaining ingredients except blueberries.
3. Now, add in the flour mixture and mix until just combined.
4. Fold in the blueberries.
5. Set the temperature of Air Fryer to 355 degrees F. Grease 12 muffin molds.
6. Put the mixture evenly into the prepared muffin molds. Arrange the molds into an Air Fryer basket.
7. Air Fry for about 12 minutes or until a toothpick inserted in the center comes out clean.
8. Remove the muffin molds from Air Fryer and place onto a wire rack to cool for about 10 minutes.
9. Carefully, invert the muffins onto the wire rack to completely cool before serving.
10. Serve.

21. Cream Breakfast Tofu

Servings: 4

Cooking Time:35 Minutes
Ingredients:
- 1 block firm tofu; pressed and cubed
- 1 tsp. rice vinegar
- 2 tbsp. soy sauce
- 1 tbsp. potato starch
- 2 tsp. sesame oil
- 1 cup Greek yogurt

Directions:
1. In a bowl; mix tofu cubes with vinegar, soy sauce and oil, toss, and leave aside for 15 minutes.
2. Dip tofu cubes in potato starch, toss, transfer to your air fryer; heat up at 370 °F and cook for 20 minutes shaking halfway. Divide into bowls and serve for breakfast with some Greek yogurt on the side.

22. Peanut Butter Bread

Servings: 3
Cooking Time: 15 Minutes
Ingredients:
- 1 tbsp. oil
- 2 tbsp. peanut butter
- 4 slices bread
- 1 banana, sliced

Directions:
1. Spread the peanut butter on top of each slice of bread, then arrange the banana slices on top. Sandwich two slices together, then the other two.
2. Oil the inside of the Air Fryer and cook the bread for 5 minutes at 300°F.

23. Fish Sticks

Servings: 4
Cooking Time: 10 Minutes
Ingredients:
- 8 oz cod fillet
- 1 egg, beaten
- ¼ cup coconut flour
- ¼ teaspoon ground coriander
- ¼ teaspoon ground paprika
- ¼ teaspoon ground cumin
- ¼ teaspoon Pink salt
- 1/3 cup coconut flakes
- 1 tablespoon mascarpone
- 1 teaspoon heavy cream
- Cooking spray

Directions:
1. Chop the cod fillet roughly and put it in the blender. Add egg, coconut flour ground coriander, paprika, cumin, salt, and blend the mixture until smooth. After this, transfer it in the bowl. Line the chopping board with parchment. Place the fish mixture over the parchment and flatten it in the shape of the flat square. Then cut the fish square into sticks. In the separated bowl whisk together heavy cream and mascarpone. Sprinkle every fish stick with mascarpone mixture and after this coat in the coconut flakes. Preheat the air fryer to 400F. Spray the air fryer basket with cooking spray and arrange the fish sticks inside. Cook the fish sticks for 10 minutes. Flip them on another side in halfway of cooking.

24. Scallion Eggs Bake

Servings: 2
Cooking Time: 20 Minutes
Ingredients:
- 2 eggs
- 4 oz double Gloucester cheese, grated'
- 1 teaspoon coconut flour
- ¼ cup heavy cream
- 1 tablespoon butter
- 1 tablespoon scallions, chopped

Directions:
1. Place the eggs on the rack and insert the rack in the air fryer. Cook the eggs for 17 minutes at 250F. Then cool the eggs n cold water and peel. Cut the eggs into halves. In the bowl mix up cheese, heavy cream, butter, and coconut flour. Microwave the mixture for 1 minute or until it is liquid. Place the egg halves in the 2 ramekins. Pour the cheese mixture over the eggs and top with scallions. Place the ramekins in the air fryer and cook them for 3 minutes at 400F.

25. Sausage Quiche

Servings: 4
Cooking Time: 35 Minutes
Ingredients:
- 12 large eggs
- 1 cup heavy cream
- 1 tsp black pepper
- 12 oz sugar-free breakfast sausage
- 2 cups shredded cheddar cheese

Directions:
1. Preheat your fryer to 375°F/190°C.
2. In a large bowl, whisk the eggs, heavy cream, salad and pepper together.
3. Add the breakfast sausage and cheddar cheese.
4. Pour the mixture into a greased casserole dish.
5. Bake for 25 minutes.
6. Cut into 12 squares and serve hot.

26. Crust-less Quiche

Servings:2
Cooking Time:30 Minutes
Ingredients:
- 4 eggs
- ¼ cup onion, chopped

- ½ cup tomatoes, chopped
- ½ cup milk
- 1 cup Gouda cheese, shredded
- Salt, to taste

Directions:
1. Preheat the Air fryer to 340 °F and grease 2 ramekins lightly.
2. Mix together all the ingredients in a ramekin until well combined.
3. Place in the Air fryer and cook for about 30 minutes.
4. Dish out and serve.

27. Grilled Beef Steak With Herby Marinade

Servings:2
Cooking Time: 40 Minutes
Ingredients:
- 2 porterhouse steaks
- Salt and pepper to taste
- ¼ cup fish sauce
- 2 tablespoons marjoram
- 2 tablespoons thyme
- 2 tablespoons sage

Directions:
1. Place all ingredients in a Ziploc bag and allow to marinate in the fridge for at least 2 hours.
2. Preheat the air fryer at 390°F.
3. Place the grill pan accessory in the air fryer.
4. Grill for 20 minutes per batch.
5. Flip every 10 minutes for even grilling.

28. Cheese Stuff Peppers

Servings: 8
Cooking Time: 8 Minutes
Ingredients:
- 8 small bell pepper, cut the top of peppers
- 3.5 oz feta cheese, cubed
- 1 tbsp olive oil
- 1 tsp Italian seasoning
- 1 tbsp parsley, chopped
- ¼ tsp garlic powder
- Pepper
- Salt

Directions:
1. In a bowl, toss cheese with oil and seasoning.
2. Stuff cheese in each bell peppers and place into the air fryer basket.
3. Cook at 400 F for 8 minutes.
4. Serve and enjoy.

29. Cheese Sandwich

Servings: 2
Cooking Time: 3 Minutes
Ingredients:
- 2 low carb tortillas
- 2 Cheddar cheese slices
- 2 deli ham slices
- 2 lettuce leaves
- 2 teaspoons mascarpone
- ¼ teaspoon chives, chopped

Directions:
1. Cut every tortilla into halves. In the shallow bowl mix up chives and mascarpone. Spread the tortilla halves with mascarpone mixture. Then place cheese and ham on 2 tortilla halves. Add leaves and top them with remaining tortilla halves. Preheat the air fryer to 400F. Place the tortilla sandwiches in the air fryer and cook them for 3 minutes at 400F.

30. Healthy Mix Vegetables

Servings: 4
Cooking Time: 18 Minutes
Ingredients:
- ½ cup mushrooms, sliced
- 1 onion, sliced
- ½ cup zucchini, sliced
- ½ cup squash, sliced
- ½ cup baby carrot
- 1 cup cauliflower florets
- 1 cup broccoli florets
- ¼ cup parmesan cheese
- 1 tsp red pepper flakes
- 1 tbsp garlic, minced
- 1 tbsp olive oil
- ¼ cup vinegar
- ¼ tsp pepper
- ½ tsp sea salt

Directions:
1. Preheat the air fryer to 400 F.
2. In a bowl, mix together oil, vinegar, garlic, pepper, red pepper flakes, and salt.
3. Add vegetables into the bowl and toss to coat.
4. Transfer vegetable mixture into the air fryer basket and cook for 16 minutes. Shake basket halfway through.
5. Sprinkle with cheese and cook for 1-2 minutes more.
6. Serve and enjoy.

31. Vegetable Quiche

Servings: 6
Cooking Time: 24 Minutes
Ingredients:
- 8 eggs
- 1 cup coconut milk
- 1 cup tomatoes, chopped
- 1 cup zucchini, chopped
- 1 tbsp butter
- 1 onion, chopped
- 1 cup Parmesan cheese, grated
- 1/2 tsp pepper
- 1 tsp salt

Directions:
1. Preheat the air fryer to 370 F.
2. Melt butter in a pan over medium heat then add onion and sauté until onion lightly brown.
3. Add tomatoes and zucchini to the pan and sauté for 4-5 minutes.
4. Transfer cooked vegetables into the air fryer baking dish.
5. Beat eggs with cheese, milk, pepper, and salt in a bowl.
6. Pour egg mixture over vegetables in a baking dish.
7. Place dish in the air fryer and cook for 24 minutes or until eggs are set.
8. Slice and serve.

32. Cheddar Turkey Casserole

Servings: 4
Cooking Time: 25 Minutes
Ingredients:
- 1 turkey breast, skinless, boneless, cut into strips and browned
- 2 teaspoons olive oil
- 2 cups almond milk
- 2 cups cheddar cheese, shredded
- 2 eggs, whisked
- Salt and black pepper to the taste
- 1 tablespoon chives, chopped

Directions:
1. In a bowl, mix the eggs with milk, cheese, salt, pepper and the chives and whisk well. Preheat the air fryer at 330 degrees F, add the oil, heat it up, add the turkey pieces and spread them well. Add the eggs mixture, toss a bit and cook for 25 minutes. Serve right away for breakfast.

33. Zucchini Omelet

Servings:2
Cooking Time: 14 Minutes
Ingredients:
- 1 teaspoon butter
- 1 zucchini, julienned
- 4 eggs
- ¼ teaspoon fresh basil, chopped
- ¼ teaspoon red pepper flakes, crushed
- Salt and ground black pepper, as required

Directions:
1. Set the temperature of Air Fryer to 355 degrees F. Grease an Air Fryer pan.
2. Take a skillet, melt the butter over medium heat and cook the zucchini for about 3-4 minutes.
3. Meanwhile, in a bowl, mix together the eggs, basil, red pepper flakes, salt, and black pepper.
4. Add the cooked zucchini and gently, stir to combine.

5. Transfer the mixture into the prepared pan.
6. Air Fry for 10 minutes or until done completely.
7. Serve hot.

34. Chia And Hemp Pudding

Servings: 2
Cooking Time: 2 Minutes
Ingredients:
- 1 teaspoon hemp seeds
- 1 teaspoon chia seeds
- 1 tablespoon almond flour
- 1 teaspoon coconut flakes
- 1 teaspoon walnuts, chopped
- ½ teaspoon flax meal
- ¼ teaspoon vanilla extract
- ½ teaspoon Erythritol
- ½ cup of coconut milk
- ¼ cup water, boiled

Directions:
1. Put hemp seeds, chia seeds, almond flour, coconut flakes, walnuts, flax meal, vanilla extract, coconut milk, and water in the big bowl. Stir the mixture until homogenous and pour it into 2 mason jars. Leave the mason jars in the cold place for 4 hours. Then top the surface of the pudding with Erythritol. Place the mason jars in the air fryer and cook the pudding for 2 minutes at 400F or until you get the light brown crust.

35. Perfect Breakfast Frittata(2)

Servings: 2
Cooking Time: 10 Minutes
Ingredients:
- 2 large eggs
- 1 tbsp bell peppers, chopped
- 1 tbsp spring onions, chopped
- 1 sausage patty, chopped
- 1 tbsp butter, melted
- 2 tbsp cheddar cheese
- Pepper
- Salt

Directions:
1. Add sausage patty in air fryer baking dish and cook in air fryer 350 F for 5 minutes.
2. Meanwhile, in a bowl whisk together eggs, pepper, and salt.
3. Add bell peppers, onions and stir well.
4. Pour egg mixture over sausage patty and stir well.
5. Sprinkle with cheese and cook in the air fryer at 350 F for 5 minutes.
6. Serve and enjoy.

36. Bacon Eggs

Servings: 2
Cooking Time: 5 Minutes
Ingredients:

- 2 eggs, hard-boiled, peeled
- 4 bacon slices
- ½ teaspoon avocado oil
- 1 teaspoon mustard

Directions:
1. Preheat the air fryer to 400F. Then sprinkle the air fryer basket with avocado oil and place the bacon slices inside. Flatten them in one layer and cook for 2 minutes from each side. After this, cool the bacon to the room temperature. Wrap every egg into 2 bacon slices. Secure the eggs with toothpicks and place them in the air fryer. Cook the wrapped eggs for 1 minute at 400F.

37. Egg & Mushroom Scramble

Servings:2
Cooking Time: 10 Minutes
Ingredients:
- 4 eggs
- Salt and freshly ground black pepper, as needed
- 2 tablespoons unsalted butter
- ½ cup fresh mushrooms, finely chopped
- 2 tablespoons Parmesan cheese, shredded

Directions:
1. Set the temperature of Air Fryer to 285 degrees F.
2. In a bowl, mix together the eggs, salt, and black pepper.
3. In a baking pan, melt the butter and tilt the pan to spread the butter in the bottom.
4. Add the beaten eggs and Air Fry for about 4-5 minutes
5. Add in the mushrooms and cheese and cook for 5 minutes, stirring occasionally.
6. Serve hot.

38. Jalapeno Breakfast Muffins

Servings: 8
Cooking Time: 15 Minutes
Ingredients:
- 5 eggs
- 1/3 cup coconut oil, melted
- 2 tsp baking powder
- 3 tbsp erythritol
- 3 tbsp jalapenos, sliced
- 1/4 cup unsweetened coconut milk
- 2/3 cup coconut flour
- 3/4 tsp sea salt

Directions:
1. Preheat the air fryer to 325 F.
2. In a large bowl, stir together coconut flour, baking powder, erythritol, and sea salt.
3. Stir in eggs, jalapenos, coconut milk, and coconut oil until well combined.
4. Pour batter into the silicone muffin molds and place into the air fryer basket.

5. Cook muffins for 15 minutes.
6. Serve and enjoy.

39. Pea Delight

Servings: 2 – 4
Cooking Time: 25 Minutes
Ingredients:
- 1 cup flour
- 1 tsp. baking powder
- 3 eggs
- 1 cup coconut milk
- 1 cup cream cheese
- 3 tbsp. pea protein
- ½ cup chicken/turkey strips
- 1 pinch sea salt
- 1 cup mozzarella cheese

Directions:
1. Set your Air Fryer at 390°F and allow to warm.
2. In a large bowl, mix all ingredients together using a large wooden spoon.
3. Spoon equal amounts of the mixture into muffin cups and allow to cook for 15 minutes.

40. Prosciutto & Mozzarella Bruschetta

Servings:1
Cooking Time: 7 Minutes
Ingredients:
- 3 oz chopped mozzarella
- 3 prosciutto slices, chopped
- 1 tbsp olive oil
- 1 tsp dried basil
- 6 small slices of French bread

Directions:
1. Preheat the air fryer to 350 F. Place the bread slices and toast for 3 minutes. Top the bread with tomatoes, prosciutto and mozzarella.
2. Sprinkle the basil over the mozzarella. Drizzle with olive oil. Return to the air fryer and cook for 1 more minute, enough to become melty and warm.

41. Homemade Crispy Croutons

Servings:4
Cooking Time: 20 Minutes
Ingredients:
- 2 tbsp butter, melted
- Garlic salt and black pepper to taste

Directions:
1. Mix bread with butter, garlic salt, and pepper until well-coated. Place in the air fryer, cook for 12 minutes at 380 F until golden brown and crispy.

42. Egg In A Bread Basket

Servings:2
Cooking Time:10 Minutes

Ingredients:

- 2 bread slices
- 1 bacon slice, chopped
- 4 tomato slices
- 1 tablespoon Mozzarella cheese, shredded
- 2 eggs
- ½ tablespoon olive oil
- 1/8 teaspoon maple syrup
- 1/8 teaspoon balsamic vinegar
- ¼ teaspoon fresh parsley, chopped
- Salt and black pepper, to taste
- 2 tablespoons mayonnaise

Directions:

1. Preheat the Air fryer to 320 °F and grease 2 ramekins lightly.
2. Place 1 bread slice in each prepared ramekin and add bacon and tomato slices.
3. Top evenly with the Mozzarella cheese and crack 1 egg in each ramekin.
4. Drizzle with balsamic vinegar and maple syrup and season with parsley, salt and black pepper.
5. Arrange the ramekins in an Air fryer basket and cook for about 10 minutes.
6. Top with mayonnaise and serve immediately.

43. Mock Stir Fry

Servings:4
Cooking Time: 25 Minutes
Ingredients:

- 2 carrots, sliced
- 1 red bell pepper, cut into strips
- 1 yellow bell pepper, cut into strips
- 1 cup snow peas
- 15 oz broccoli florets
- 1 scallion, sliced
- Sauce:
- 3 tbsp soy sauce
- 2 tbsp oyster sauce
- 1 tbsp brown sugar
- 1 tsp sesame oil
- 1 tsp cornstarch
- 1 tsp sriracha
- 2 garlic cloves, minced
- 1 tbsp grated ginger
- 1 tbsp rice wine vinegar

Directions:

1. Preheat the air fryer to 370 F. Place the chicken, bell peppers, and carrot, in a bowl. In another bowl, combine the sauce ingredients. Coat the chicken mixture with the sauce.
2. Place on a lined baking sheet and cook for 5 minutes. Add snow peas and broccoli and cook for an additional 8 to 10 minutes. Serve garnished with scallion.

44. Turmeric Mozzarella Sticks

Servings: 2
Cooking Time: 7 Minutes
Ingredients:

- 4 oz Mozzarella
- 2 tablespoons coconut flakes
- 1 egg, beaten
- 1 teaspoon turmeric powder
- 1 tablespoon heavy cream
- ½ teaspoon ground black pepper
- Cooking spray

Directions:

1. Cut Mozzarella into 2 sticks. Then in the mixing bowl mix up heavy cream, egg, and ground black pepper. Dip the cheese sticks in the liquid. After this, coat every cheese stick with coconut flakes. Preheat the air fryer to 400F. Then spray the air fryer basket with cooking spray. Put Mozzarella sticks in the air fryer and cook them for 7 minutes or until they are light brown.

45. Choco Bread

Servings: 12
Cooking Time: 30 Minutes
Ingredients:

- 1 tbsp. flax egg [1 tbsp. flax meal + 3 tbsp. water]
- 1 cup zucchini, shredded and squeezed
- ½ cup sunflower oil
- ½ cup maple syrup
- 1 tsp. vanilla extract
- 1 tsp. apple cider vinegar
- ½ cup milk
- 1 cup flour
- 1 tsp. baking soda
- ½ cup unsweetened cocoa powder
- ¼ tsp. salt
- ⅓ cup chocolate chips

Directions:

1. Pre-heat your Air Fryer to 350°F.
2. Take a baking dish small enough to fit inside the fryer and line it with parchment paper.
3. Mix together the flax meal, zucchini, sunflower oil, maple, vanilla, apple cider vinegar and milk in a bowl.
4. Incorporate the flour, cocoa powder, salt and baking soda, stirring all the time to combine everything well.
5. Finally, throw in the chocolate chips.
6. Transfer the batter to the baking dish and cook in the fryer for 15 minutes. Make sure to test with a toothpick before serving by sticking it in the center. The bread is ready when the toothpick comes out clean.

46. Spicy Egg And Bacon Wraps

Servings:3

Cooking Time: 15 Minutes
Ingredients:
- 2 previously scrambled eggs
- 3 slices bacon, cut into strips
- 3 tbsp salsa
- 3 tbsp cream cheese, divided
- 1 cup grated pepper Jack cheese

Directions:
1. Preheat air fryer to 390 F. Spread cream cheese onto tortillas. Divide the eggs and bacon between the tortillas. Top with salsa. Sprinkle some grated cheese over. Roll up the tortillas. Cook for 10 minutes.

47. Bistro Wedges

Servings: 4
Cooking Time: 20 Minutes
Ingredients:
- 1 lb. fingerling potatoes, cut into wedges
- 1 tsp. extra virgin olive oil
- ½ tsp. garlic powder
- Salt and pepper to taste
- ½ cup raw cashews, soaked in water overnight
- ½ tsp. ground turmeric
- ½ tsp. paprika
- 1 tbsp. nutritional yeast
- 1 tsp. fresh lemon juice
- 2 tbsp. to ¼ cup water

Directions:
1. Pre-heat your Air Fryer at 400°F.
2. In a bowl, toss together the potato wedges, olive oil, garlic powder, and salt and pepper, making sure to coat the potatoes well.
3. Transfer the potatoes to the basket of your fryer and fry for 10 minutes.
4. In the meantime, prepare the cheese sauce. Pulse the cashews, turmeric, paprika, nutritional yeast, lemon juice, and water together in a food processor. Add more water to achieve your desired consistency.
5. When the potatoes are finished cooking, move them to a bowl that is small enough to fit inside the fryer and add the cheese sauce on top. Cook for an additional 3 minutes.

48. Onion And Cheese Omelet

Servings:1
Cooking Time: 15 Minutes
Ingredients:
- 2 tbsp grated cheddar cheese
- 1 tsp soy sauce
- ½ onion, sliced
- ¼ tsp pepper
- 1 tbsp olive oil

Directions:
1. Whisk the eggs along with the pepper and soy sauce. Preheat the air fryer to 350 F. Heat the olive oil and add the egg mixture

and the onion. Cook for 8 to 10 minutes. Top with the grated cheddar cheese.

49. Mushroom Cheese Salad

Servings: 3
Cooking Time: 15 Minutes
Ingredients:
- 10 mushrooms, halved
- 1 tbsp fresh parsley, chopped
- 1 tbsp olive oil
- 1 tbsp mozzarella cheese, grated
- 1 tbsp cheddar cheese, grated
- 1 tbsp dried mix herbs
- Pepper
- Salt

Directions:
1. Add all ingredients into the bowl and toss well.
2. Transfer bowl mixture into the air fryer baking dish.
3. Place in the air fryer and cook at 380 F for 15 minutes.
4. Serve and enjoy.

50. Potato & Kale Nuggets

Servings: 4
Cooking Time: 25 Minutes
Ingredients:
- 1 tsp. extra virgin olive oil
- 1 clove of garlic, minced
- 4 cups kale, rinsed and chopped
- 2 cups potatoes, boiled and mashed
- 1/8 cup milk
- Salt and pepper to taste
- Vegetable oil

Directions:
1. Pre-heat your Air Fryer at 390°F.
2. In a skillet over medium heat, fry the garlic in the olive oil, until it turns golden brown. Cook with the kale for an additional 3 minutes and remove from the heat.
3. Mix the mashed potatoes, kale and garlic in a bowl. Throw in the milk and sprinkle with some salt and pepper as desired.
4. Shape the mixture into nuggets and spritz each one with a little vegetable oil. Put in the basket of your fryer and leave to cook for 15 minutes, shaking the basket halfway through cooking to make sure the nuggets fry evenly.

51. Perfect Cheesy Eggs

Servings:2
Cooking Time:12 Minutes
Ingredients:
- 2 teaspoons unsalted butter, softened
- 2-ounce ham, sliced thinly
- 4 large eggs, divided

- 3 tablespoons Parmesan cheese, grated finely
- 2 teaspoons fresh chives, minced
- 2 tablespoons heavy cream
- 1/8 teaspoon smoked paprika
- Salt and black pepper, to taste

Directions:
1. Preheat the Air fryer to 320 °F and grease a pie pan with butter.
2. Whisk together 1 egg with cream, salt and black pepper in a bowl.
3. Place ham slices in the bottom of the pie pan and top with the egg mixture.
4. Crack the remaining eggs on top and season with smoked paprika, salt and black pepper.
5. Top evenly with Parmesan cheese and chives and transfer the pie pan in the Air fryer.
6. Cook for about 12 minutes and serve with toasted bread slices.

52. Buttered Eggs In Hole

Servings:2
Cooking Time: 11 Minutes
Ingredients:
- 2 eggs
- Salt and pepper to taste
- 2 tbsp butter

Directions:
1. Place a heatproof bowl in the fryer's basket and brush with butter. Make a hole in the middle of the bread slices with a bread knife and place in the heatproof bowl in 2 batches. Break an egg into the center of each hole. Season with salt and pepper. Close the air fryer and cook for 4 minutes at 330 F. Turn the bread with a spatula and cook for another 4 minutes. Serve as a breakfast accompaniment.

53. Breakfast Omelet

Servings: 2
Cooking Time: 30 Minutes
Ingredients:
- 1 large onion, chopped
- 2 tbsp. cheddar cheese, grated
- 3 eggs
- ½ tsp. soy sauce
- Salt
- Pepper powder
- Cooking spray

Directions:
1. In a bowl, mix the salt, pepper powder, soy sauce and eggs with a whisk.
2. Take a small pan small enough to fit inside the Air Fryer and spritz with cooking spray. Spread the chopped onion across the bottom of the pan, then transfer the pan to

the Fryer. Cook at 355°F for 6-7 minutes, ensuring the onions turn translucent.
3. Add the egg mixture on top of the onions, coating everything well. Add the cheese on top, then resume cooking for another 5 or 6 minutes.
4. Take care when taking the pan out of the fryer. Enjoy with some toasted bread.

54. Almond Crust Chicken

Servings: 2
Cooking Time: 25 Minutes
Ingredients:
- 2 chicken breasts, skinless and boneless
- 1 tbsp Dijon mustard
- 2 tbsp mayonnaise
- ¼ cup almonds
- Pepper
- Salt

Directions:
1. Add almond into the food processor and process until finely ground. Transfer almonds on a plate and set aside.
2. Mix together mustard and mayonnaise and spread over chicken.
3. Coat chicken with almond and place into the air fryer basket and cook at 350 F for 25 minutes.
4. Serve and enjoy.

55. Indian Cauliflower

Servings: 2
Cooking Time: 20 Minutes
Ingredients:
- 3 cups cauliflower florets
- 2 tbsp water
- 2 tsp fresh lemon juice
- ½ tbsp ginger paste
- 1 tsp chili powder
- ¼ tsp turmeric
- ½ cup vegetable stock
- Pepper
- Salt

Directions:
1. Add all ingredients into the air fryer baking dish and mix well.
2. Place dish in the air fryer and cook at 400 F for 10 minutes.
3. Stir well and cook at 360 F for 10 minutes more.
4. Stir well and serve.

56. Egg Veggie Frittata

Servings:2
Cooking Time:13 Minutes
Ingredients:
- 4 eggs
- ½ cup milk
- 2 green onions, chopped

- ¼ cup baby Bella mushrooms, chopped
- ¼ cup spinach, chopped
- ½ teaspoon salt
- ½ teaspoon black pepper
- Dash of hot sauce

Directions:
1. Preheat the Air fryer to 365 °F and grease 6x3 inch square pan with butter.
2. Whisk eggs with milk in a large bowl and stir in green onions, mushrooms and spinach.
3. Sprinkle with salt, black pepper and hot sauce and pour this mixture into the prepared pan.
4. Place in the Air fryer and cook for about 18 minutes.
5. Dish out in a platter and serve warm.

57. Chocolate Banana Bread

Servings:10
Cooking Time: 20 Minutes
Ingredients:
- 2 cups flour
- ½ teaspoon baking soda
- ½ teaspoon baking powder
- ½ teaspoon salt
- ¾ cup sugar
- 1/3 cup butter, softened
- 3 eggs
- 1 tablespoon vanilla extract
- 1 cup milk
- ½ cup bananas, peeled and mashed
- 1 cup chocolate chips

Directions:
1. Take a bowl and mix together the flour, baking soda, baking powder, and salt.
2. In another large bowl, add the butter, and sugar. Beat until light and fluffy.
3. Now, add in the eggs, and vanilla extract. Beat until well combined.
4. Add the flour mixture and mix until well combined.
5. Add in the milk, and mashed bananas and mix them well.
6. Gently, fold in the chocolate chips.
7. Set the temperature of Air Fryer to 360 degrees F. Grease a loaf pan.
8. Place the mixture evenly into the prepared pan.
9. Arrange the loaf pan into an Air Fryer basket.
10. Air Fry for about 20 minutes or until a toothpick inserted in the center comes out clean.
11. Remove from Air Fryer and place the pan onto a wire rack for about 10-15 minutes.
12. Carefully, take out the bread from pan and put onto a wire rack until it is completely cool before slicing.

13. Cut the bread into desired size slices and serve.

58. Scotch Eggs

Servings: 4
Cooking Time: 40 Minutes
Ingredients:
- 4 large eggs
- 1 package Jimmy Dean's Pork Sausage (12 oz)
- 8 slices thick-cut bacon
- 4 toothpicks

Directions:
1. Hard-boil the eggs, peel the shells and let them cool.
2. Slice the sausage into four parts and place each part into a large circle.
3. Put an egg into each circle and wrap it in the sausage.
4. Place inside your refrigerator for 1 hour.
5. Make a cross with two pieces of thick-cut bacon.
6. Place a wrapped egg in the center, fold the bacon over top of the egg and secure with a toothpick.
7. Cook inside your fryer at 450°F/230°C for 25 minutes.
8. Enjoy!

59. Sweet Rosemary Cornbread

Servings:4
Cooking Time: 25 Minutes
Ingredients:
- ¾ cup fine yellow cornmeal
- ½ cup sorghum flour
- ¼ cup tapioca starch
- ½ teaspoon xanthan gum*
- ¼ cup granulated sugar
- 2 teaspoons baking powder
- ¼ teaspoon salt
- 1 cup plain almond milk
- 3 tablespoons olive oil
- 2 teaspoons fresh rosemary, minced

Directions:
1. In a large bowl, mix together the cornmeal, sorghum flour, tapioca starch, xanthan gum, sugar, baking powder, and salt.
2. Add the almond milk, oil, and rosemary. Mix until well combined.
3. Set the temperature of Air Fryer to 400 degrees F. Grease 4 ramekins.
4. Put the mixture evenly into the prepared ramekins.
5. Place the ramekins into an Air Fryer basket.
6. Air Fry for about 20-25 minutes or until a toothpick inserted in the center comes out clean.

7. Remove from Air Fryer and place the ramekins onto a wire rack for about 10-15 minutes.
8. Carefully, invert the breads into serving plates.
9. Enjoy!

60. Luscious Scrambled Eggs

Servings:2
Cooking Time:10 Minutes
Ingredients:
- 2 tablespoons unsalted butter
- 4 eggs
- ¼ cup fresh mushrooms, chopped finely
- 2 tablespoons Parmesan cheese, shredded
- ¼ cup tomato, chopped finely
- Salt and black pepper, to taste

Directions:
1. Preheat the Air fryer at 285 °F and grease a baking pan.
2. Whisk together eggs with salt and black pepper in a bowl.
3. Melt butter in the baking pan and add whisked eggs, mushrooms, tomatoes and cheese.

4. Transfer in the Air fryer and cook for about 10 minutes.
5. Remove from the oven and serve warm.

61. Apple Oatmeal

Servings: 6
Cooking Time: 15 Minutes
Ingredients:
- 3 cups almond milk
- 2 apples, cored, peeled and chopped
- 1¼ cups steel cut oats
- ½ teaspoon cinnamon powder
- ¼ teaspoon nutmeg, ground
- ¼ teaspoon allspice, ground
- ¼ teaspoon ginger powder
- ¼ teaspoon cardamom, ground
- 2 teaspoons vanilla extract
- 2 teaspoons sugar
- Cooking spray

Directions:
1. Spray your air fryer with cooking spray, add all ingredients, and stir.
2. Cover and cook at 360 degrees F for 15 minutes.
3. Divide into bowls and serve.

LUNCH & DINNER RECIPES

62. Corn Stew

Servings: 4
Cooking Time: 15 Minutes
Ingredients:
- 2 leeks, chopped
- 2 tablespoons butter, melted
- 2 tomatoes, cubed
- 2 garlic cloves, minced
- 4 cups corn
- ¼ cup chicken stock
- 1 teaspoon olive oil
- 4 tarragon sprigs, chopped
- Salt and black pepper to taste
- 1 tablespoon chives, chopped

Directions:
1. Grease a pan with the oil, and then add all the ingredients and toss.
2. Place the pan in the fryer and cook at 370 degrees F for 15 minutes.
3. Divide the stew between bowls and serve.

63. Cauliflower

Servings: 4
Cooking Time: 20 Minutes
Ingredients:
- 1 head cauliflower, cut into florets
- 1 tbsp. extra-virgin olive oil
- 2 scallions, chopped
- 5 cloves of garlic, sliced
- 1 ½ tbsp. tamari
- 1 tbsp. rice vinegar
- ½ tsp. sugar
- 1 tbsp. sriracha

Directions:
1. Pre-heat the Air Fryer to 400°F.
2. Put the cauliflower florets in the Air Fryer and drizzle some oil over them before cooking for 10 minutes.
3. Turn the cauliflower over, throw in the onions and garlic, and stir. Cook for another 10 minutes.
4. Mix together the rest of the ingredients in a bowl.
5. Remove the cooked cauliflower from the fryer and coat it in the sauce.
6. Return to the Air Fryer and allow to cook for another 5 minutes. Enjoy with a side of rice.

64. Rosemary Chicken Stew

Servings: 4
Cooking Time: 20 Minutes
Ingredients:
- 2 cups okra
- 2 garlic cloves, minced
- 1 pound chicken breasts, skinless, boneless and cubed
- 4 tomatoes, cubed
- 1 tablespoon olive oil
- 1 teaspoon rosemary, dried
- Salt and black pepper to the taste
- 1 tablespoon parsley, chopped

Directions:
1. Heat up a pan that fits your air fryer with the oil over medium-high heat, add the chicken, garlic, rosemary, salt and pepper, toss and brown for 5 minutes. Add the remaining ingredients, toss again, place the pan in the air fryer and cook at 380 degrees F for 15 minutes more. Divide the stew into bowls and serve for lunch.

65. Baby Corn Pakodas

Servings: 5
Cooking Time: 20 Minutes
Ingredients:
- 1 cup flour
- ¼ tsp. baking soda
- ¼ tsp. salt
- ½ tsp. curry powder
- ½ tsp. red chili powder
- ¼ tsp. turmeric powder
- ¼ cup water
- 10 pc. baby corn, blanched

Directions:
1. Pre-heat the Air Fryer to 425°F.
2. Cover the Air Fryer basket with aluminum foil and coat with a light brushing of oil.
3. In a bowl, combine all ingredients save for the corn. Stir with a whisk until well combined.
4. Coat the corn in the batter and put inside the Air Fryer.
5. Cook for 8 minutes until a golden brown color is achieved.

66. Fried Potatoes

Servings: 1
Cooking Time: 55 Minutes
Ingredients:
- 1 medium russet potatoes, scrubbed and peeled
- 1 tsp. olive oil
- ¼ tsp. onion powder
- 1/8 tsp. salt
- A dollop of vegan butter
- A dollop of vegan cream cheese
- 1 tbsp. Kalamata olives
- 1 tbsp. chives, chopped

Directions:
1. Pre-heat the Air Fryer at 400°F.

2. In a bowl, coat the potatoes with the onion powder, salt, olive oil, and vegan butter.
3. Transfer to the fryer and allow to cook for 40 minutes, turning the potatoes over at the halfway point.
4. Take care when removing the potatoes from the fryer and enjoy with the vegan cream cheese, Kalamata olives and chives on top, plus any other vegan sides you desire.

67. Herbed Butter Rib Eye Steak

Servings: 4
Cooking Time: 60 Minutes
Ingredients:
- 4 ribeye steaks
- Olive oil
- ¾ tsp. dry rub
- ½ cup butter
- 1 tsp. dried basil
- 3 tbsp. lemon garlic seasoning

Directions:
1. Massage the olive oil into the steaks and your favorite dry rub. Leave aside to sit for thirty minutes.
2. In a bowl, combine the button, dried basil, and lemon garlic seasoning, then refrigerate.
3. Pre-heat the fryer at 450°F and set a rack inside. Place the steaks on top of the rack and allow to cook for fifteen minutes.
4. Remove the steaks from the fryer when cooked and serve with the herbed butter.

68. Turkey Avocado Rolls

Servings: 6
Cooking Time: 10 Minutes
Ingredients:
- 12 slices (12 oz) turkey breast
- 12 slices Swiss cheese
- 2 cups baby spinach
- 1 large avocado, cut into 12 slices
- 1 cup homemade mayonnaise (see recipe in Chapter 9)

Directions:
1. Lay out the slices of turkey breast flat and place a slice of Swiss cheese on top of each one.
2. Top each slice with 1 cup baby spinach and 3 slices of avocado.
3. Drizzle the mayonnaise on top.
4. Sprinkle each "sandwich" with lemon pepper.
5. Roll up the sandwiches and secure with toothpicks.
6. Serve immediately or refrigerate until ready to serve.

69. Okra And Peppers Casserole

Servings: 4
Cooking Time: 20 Minutes

Ingredients:
- 1 teaspoon olive oil
- 3 cups okra
- 2 red bell peppers, cubed
- Salt and black pepper to the taste
- 2 tomatoes, chopped
- 3 garlic cloves, minced
- ¼ cup keto tomato sauce
- 2 teaspoons coriander, ground
- 1 tablespoon cilantro, chopped
- ½ cup cheddar, shredded

Directions:
1. Grease a heat proof dish that fits your air fryer with the oil, add all the ingredients except the cilantro and the cheese and toss them really gently. Sprinkle the cheese and the cilantro on top, introduce the dish in the fryer and cook at 390 degrees F for 20 minutes. Divide between plates and serve for lunch.

70. Pork Stew

Servings: 4
Cooking Time: 25 Minutes
Ingredients:
- 1 and ½ pound pork stew meat, cubed
- ½ cup cilantro, chopped
- ½ cup green onions, chopped
- ½ cup keto tomato sauce
- A drizzle of olive oil
- 2 teaspoons chili powder

Directions:
1. Heat up a pan that fits the air fryer with the oil over medium-high heat, add the meat and brown for 5 minutes. Add the rest of the ingredients, toss, introduce the pan in the air fryer and cook at 370 degrees F for 20 minutes. Divide into and serve for lunch

71. Parmesan Beef Mix

Servings: 4
Cooking Time: 20 Minutes
Ingredients:
- 14 ounces beef, cubed
- 7 ounces keto tomato sauce
- 1 tablespoon chives, chopped
- 2 tablespoons parmesan cheese, grated
- 1 tablespoon oregano, chopped
- 1 tablespoon olive oil
- Salt and black pepper to the taste

Directions:
1. Grease a pan that fits the air fryer with the oil and mix all the ingredients except the parmesan. Sprinkle the parmesan on top, put the pan in the machine and cook at 380 degrees F for 20 minutes. Divide between plates and serve for lunch.

72. Bacon-wrapped Hot Dog

Servings: 4
Cooking Time: 25 Minutes
Ingredients:
- 4 slices sugar-free bacon
- 4 beef hot dogs

Directions:
1. Take a slice of bacon and wrap it around the hot dog, securing it with a toothpick. Repeat with the other pieces of bacon and hot dogs, placing each wrapped dog in the basket of your fryer.
2. Cook at 370°F for ten minutes, turning halfway through to fry the other side.
3. Once hot and crispy, the hot dogs are ready to serve. Enjoy!

73. Christmas Brussels Sprouts

Servings: 2
Cooking Time: 20 Minutes
Ingredients:
- 2 cups Brussels sprouts, halved
- 1 tbsp. olive oil
- 1 tbsp. balsamic vinegar
- 1 tbsp. maple syrup
- ¼ tsp. sea salt

Directions:
1. Pre-heat the Air Fryer at 375°F.
2. Evenly coat the Brussels sprouts with the olive oil, balsamic vinegar, maple syrup, and salt.
3. Transfer to the basket of your fryer and cook for 5 minutes. Give the basket a good shake, turn the heat up to 400°F and continue to cook for another 8 minutes.

74. Garlic Pork Stew

Servings: 4
Cooking Time: 30 Minutes
Ingredients:
- 1 and ½ pounds pork stew meat, cubed
- 1 red cabbage, shredded
- 1 tablespoon olive oil
- Salt and black pepper to the taste
- 2 chili peppers, chopped
- 4 garlic cloves, minced
- ½ cup veggie stock
- ¼ cup keto tomato sauce

Directions:
1. Heat up a pan that fits the air fryer with the oil over medium heat, add the meat, chili peppers and the garlic, stir and brown for 5 minutes. Add the rest of the ingredients, toss, introduce the pan in the fryer and cook at 380 degrees F for 20 minutes. Divide the into bowls and serve for lunch.

75. Falafel

Servings: 8
Cooking Time: 30 Minutes
Ingredients:
- 1 tsp. cumin seeds
- ½ tsp. coriander seeds
- 2 cups chickpeas from can, drained and rinsed
- ½ tsp. red pepper flakes
- 3 cloves garlic
- ¼ cup parsley, chopped
- ¼ cup coriander, chopped
- ½ onion, diced
- 1 tbsp. juice from freshly squeezed lemon
- 3 tbsp. flour
- ½ tsp. salt cooking spray

Directions:
1. Fry the cumin and coriander seeds over medium heat until fragrant.
2. Grind using a mortar and pestle.
3. Put all of ingredients, except for the cooking spray, in a food processor and blend until a fine consistency is achieved.
4. Use your hands to mold the mixture into falafels and spritz with the cooking spray.
5. Preheat your Air Fryer at 400°F.
6. Transfer the falafels to the fryer in one single layer.
7. Cook for 15 minutes, serving when they turn golden brown.

76. Parmesan Chicken

Servings: 4
Cooking Time: 30 Minutes
Ingredients:
- 1 teaspoon olive oil
- 4 spring onions, chopped
- 2 chicken breasts, skinless, boneless and cubed
- Salt and black pepper to the taste
- 1 and ½ cups parmesan cheese, grated
- ½ cup keto tomato sauce

Directions:
1. Preheat your air fryer at 400 degrees F, add half of the oil and the spring onions and fry them for 8 minutes, shaking the fryer halfway. Add the rest of the ingredients, toss, cook at 370 degrees F for 22 minutes, shaking the fryer halfway as well. Divide between plates and serve for lunch.

77. Pork And Spinach Stew

Servings: 4
Cooking Time: 25 Minutes
Ingredients:
- 1 pound pork stew meat, cubed
- 3 garlic cloves, minced
- ¼ cup keto tomato sauce
- 1 cup spinach, torn
- ½ teaspoon olive oil

Directions:

1. In pan that fits your air fryer, mix the pork with the other ingredients except the spinach, toss, introduce in the fryer and cook at 370 degrees F for 15 minutes. Add the spinach, toss, cook for 10 minutes more, divide into bowls and serve for lunch.

78. Pita Bread Pizza

Servings: 1
Cooking Time: 15 Minutes
Ingredients:

- 1 friendly pita bread
- 1 tbsp. pizza sauce
- 6 pepperoni slices
- ¼ cup grated mozzarella cheese
- 1 tsp. olive oil
- ¼ tsp. garlic powder
- ¼ tsp. dried oregano

Directions:

1. Pre-heat your Air Fryer to 350°F.
2. Spread the pizza sauce on top of the pita bread. Place the pepperoni slices over the sauce, followed by the mozzarella cheese.
3. Season with garlic powder and oregano.
4. Put the pita pizza inside the Air Fryer and place a trivet on top.
5. Cook for 6 minutes and enjoy.

79. Potatoes And Calamari Stew

Servings: 4
Cooking Time: 16 Minutes
Ingredients:

- 10 ounces calamari, cut into strips
- 1 cup red wine
- 1 cup water
- 2 tablespoons olive oil
- 2 teaspoons pepper sauce
- 1 tablespoon hot sauce
- 1 tablespoon sweet paprika
- 1 tablespoon tomato sauce
- Salt and black pepper to taste
- ½ bunch cilantro, chopped
- 2 garlic cloves, minced
- 1 yellow onion, chopped
- 4 potatoes, cut into quarters.

Directions:

1. Place all the ingredients in a pan that fits the air fryer and toss.
2. Put the pan in the fryer and cook at 400 degrees F for 16 minutes.
3. Divide the stew between bowls and serve.

80. Cauliflower Rice Chicken Curry

Servings: 4
Cooking Time: 40 Minutes
Ingredients:

- 2 lb chicken (4 breasts)
- 1 packet curry paste
- 3 tbsp ghee (can substitute with butter)

- ½ cup heavy cream
- 1 head cauliflower (around 1 kg/2.2 lb)

Directions:

1. Melt the ghee in a pot. Mix in the curry paste.
2. Add the water and simmer for 5 minutes.
3. Add the chicken, cover, and simmer on a medium heat for 20 minutes or until the chicken is cooked.
4. Shred the cauliflower florets in a food processor to resemble rice.
5. Once the chicken is cooked, uncover, and incorporate the cream.
6. Cook for 7 minutes and serve over the cauliflower.

81. Chicken And Pepper Mix

Servings: 6
Cooking Time: 20 Minutes
Ingredients:

- 3-pound chicken breast, skinless, boneless
- 1 tablespoon tikka seasonings
- 1 tomato, roughly chopped
- 1 green bell pepper, roughly chopped
- 1 tablespoon coconut oil
- 2 spring onions, chopped

Directions:

1. Chop the chicken breast roughly and put it in the mixing bowl. Add tikka seasonings, bell pepper, and spring onion. Mix up the ingredients and leave for 10 minutes to marinate. Then preheat the air fryer to 360F. Put the chicken mixture and tomatoes in the air fryer basket. Cook the chicken tikkas for 20 minutes.

82. Roast Beef Lettuce Wraps

Servings: 4
Cooking Time: 10 Minutes
Ingredients:

- 8 large iceberg lettuce leaves
- 8 oz (8 slices) rare roast beef
- ½ cup homemade mayonnaise
- 8 slices provolone cheese
- 1 cup baby spinach

Directions:

1. Wash the lettuce leaves and sake them dry. Try not to rip them.
2. Place 1 slice of roast beef inside each wrap.
3. Smother 1 tablespoon of mayonnaise on top of each piece of roast beef.
4. Top the mayonnaise with 1 slice of provolone cheese and 1 cup of baby spinach.
5. Roll the lettuce up around the toppings.
6. Serve & enjoy!

83. Mashed Garlic Turnips

Servings: 2
Cooking Time: 10 Minutes

Ingredients:
- 3 cups diced turnip
- 2 cloves garlic, minced
- ¼ cup heavy cream
- 3 tbsp melted butter
- Salt and pepper to season

Directions:
1. Boil the turnips until tender.
2. Drain and mash the turnips.
3. Add the cream, butter, salt, pepper and garlic. Combine well.
4. Serve!

84. Chicken Stew

Servings: 6
Cooking Time: 30 Minutes
Ingredients:
- 1 tablespoon butter, soft
- 4 celery stalks, chopped
- 2 red bell peppers, chopped
- 1 pound chicken breasts, skinless, boneless and cubed
- 2 teaspoons garlic, minced
- Salt and black pepper to the taste
- ½ cup coconut cream

Directions:
1. Grease a baking dish that fits your air fryer with the butter, add all the ingredients in the pan and toss them. Introduce the dish in the fryer, cook at 360 degrees F for 30 minutes, divide into bowls and serve for lunch.

85. Rosemary Rib Eye Steaks

Servings: 2
Cooking Time: 40 Minutes
Ingredients:
- ¼ cup butter
- 1 clove minced garlic
- Salt and pepper
- 1 ½ tbsp. balsamic vinegar
- ¼ cup rosemary, chopped
- 2 ribeye steaks

Directions:
1. Melt the butter in a skillet over medium heat. Add the garlic and fry until fragrant.
2. Remove the skillet from the heat and add in the salt, pepper, and vinegar. Allow it to cool.
3. Add the rosemary, then pour the whole mixture into a Ziploc bag.
4. Put the ribeye steaks in the bag and shake well, making sure to coat the meat well. Refrigerate for an hour, then allow to sit for a further twenty minutes.
5. Pre-heat the fryer at 400°F and set the rack inside. Cook the ribeyes for fifteen minutes.
6. Take care when removing the steaks from the fryer and plate up. Enjoy!

86. Stuffed Avocado

Servings: 2
Cooking Time: 10 Minutes
Ingredients:
- 1 avocado, peeled, pitted
- 2 tablespoons coconut flour
- 1 egg, beaten
- 1 tablespoon pork rinds, grinded
- 1 oz ground pork
- 1 oz Parmesan, grated
- 1 teaspoon avocado oil
- Cooking spray

Directions:
1. Heat up the skillet on the medium heat and add avocado oil. Add ground pork and cook it for 3 minutes. Stir it from time to time to avoid burning. Then add grated cheese and stir the mixture until cheese is melted. Remove the mixture from the heat. After this, fill the avocado with the ground pork mixture and pork rinds. Secure two halves of avocado together and dip in the egg. Then coat the avocado in the coconut four and dip in the egg again. After this, coat the avocado in the coconut flour one more time. Preheat the air fryer to 400F. Place the avocado bomb in the air fryer and spray it with cooking spray. Cook the meal for 6 minutes at 400F. Cut the cooked avocado bomb into 2 servings and transfer in the serving plate.

87. Mu Shu Lunch Pork

Servings: 2
Cooking Time: 10 Minutes
Ingredients:
- 4 cups coleslaw mix, with carrots
- 1 small onion, sliced thin
- 1 lb cooked roast pork, cut into ½" cubes
- 2 tbsp hoisin sauce
- 2 tbsp soy sauce

Directions:
1. In a large skillet, heat the oil on a high heat.
2. Stir-fry the cabbage and onion for 4 minutes until tender.
3. Add the pork, hoisin and soy sauce.
4. Cook until browned.
5. Enjoy!

88. Chili Bell Peppers Stew

Servings: 4
Cooking Time: 15 Minutes
Ingredients:
- 2 red bell peppers, cut into wedges
- 2 green bell peppers, cut into wedges
- 2 yellow bell peppers, cut into wedges
- ½ cup keto tomato sauce
- 1 tablespoon chili powder
- 2 teaspoons cumin, ground
- ¼ teaspoon sweet paprika

- Salt and black pepper to the taste

Directions:
1. In a pan that fits your air fryer, mix all the ingredients, toss, introduce the pan in the machine and cook at 370 degrees F for 15 minutes. Divide into bowls and serve for lunch.

89. Tofu & Sweet Potatoes

Servings: 8
Cooking Time: 50 Minutes
Ingredients:
- 8 sweet potatoes, scrubbed
- 2 tbsp. olive oil
- 1 large onion, chopped
- 2 green chilies, deseeded and chopped
- ½ lb. tofu, crumbled
- 2 tbsp. Cajun seasoning
- cup tomatoes
- 1 can kidney beans, drained and rinsed
- Salt and pepper to taste

Directions:
1. Pre-heat the Air Fryer at 400°F.
2. With a knife, pierce the skin of the sweet potatoes in numerous places and cook in the fryer for half an hour, making sure they become soft. Remove from the fryer, halve each potato, and set to one side.
3. Over a medium heat, fry the onions and chilis in a little oil for 2 minutes until fragrant.
4. Add in the tofu and Cajun seasoning and allow to cook for a further 3 minutes before incorporating the kidney beans and tomatoes. Sprinkle some salt and pepper as desire.
5. Top each sweet potato halve with a spoonful of the tofu mixture and serve.

90. Mozzarella Beef

Servings: 6
Cooking Time: 30 Minutes
Ingredients:
- 12 oz. beef brisket
- 2 tsp. Italian herbs
- 2 tsp. butter
- 1 onion, sliced
- 7 oz. mozzarella cheese, sliced

Directions:
1. Pre-heat the fryer at 365°F.
2. Cut up the brisket into four equal slices and season with the Italian herbs.
3. Allow the butter to melt in the fryer. Place the slices of beef inside along with the onion. Put a piece of mozzarella on top of each piece of brisket and cook for twenty-five minutes.
4. Enjoy!

91. Almond Chicken Curry

Servings: 2
Cooking Time: 15 Minutes
Ingredients:
- 10 oz chicken fillet, chopped
- 1 teaspoon ground turmeric
- ½ cup spring onions, diced
- 1 teaspoon salt
- ½ teaspoon curry powder
- ½ teaspoon garlic, diced
- ½ teaspoon ground coriander
- ½ cup of organic almond milk
- 1 teaspoon Truvia
- 1 teaspoon olive oil

Directions:
1. Put the chicken in the bowl. Add the ground turmeric, salt, curry powder, diced garlic, ground coriander, and almond Truvia. Then add olive oil and mix up the chicken. After this, add almond milk and transfer the chicken in the air fryer pan. Then preheat the air fryer to 375F and place the pan with korma curry inside. Top the chicken with diced onion. Cook the meal for 10 minutes. Stir it after 5 minutes of cooking. If the chicken is not cooked after 10 minutes, cook it for an additional 5 minutes.

92. Tomato And Peppers Stew

Servings: 4
Cooking Time: 15 Minutes
Ingredients:
- 4 spring onions, chopped
- 2 pound tormatoes, cubed
- 1 teaspoon sweet paprika
- Salt and black pepper to the taste
- 2 red bell peppers, cubed
- 1 tablespoon cilantro, chopped

Directions:
1. In a pan that fits your air fryer, mix all the ingredients, toss, introduce the pan in the fryer and cook at 360 degrees F for 15 minutes. Divide into bowls and serve for lunch.

93. Chili Potato Wedges

Servings: 4
Cooking Time: 50 Minutes
Ingredients:
- 1 lb. fingerling potatoes, washed and cut into wedges
- 1 tsp. olive oil
- 1 tsp. salt
- 1 tsp. black pepper
- 1 tsp. cayenne pepper
- 1 tsp. nutritional yeast
- ½ tsp. garlic powder

Directions:

1. Pre-heat the Air Fryer at 400°F.
2. Coat the potatoes with the rest of the ingredients.
3. Transfer to the basket of your fryer and allow to cook for 16 minutes, shaking the basket at the halfway point.

94. Green Beans Stew

Servings: 4
Cooking Time: 15 Minutes
Ingredients:
- 1 pound green beans, halved
- 1 cup okra
- 1 tablespoon thyme, chopped
- 3 tablespoons keto tomato sauce
- Salt and black pepper to the taste
- 4 garlic cloves, minced

Directions:
1. In a pan that fits your air fryer, mix all the ingredients, toss, introduce the pan in the air fryer and cook at 370 degrees F for 15 minutes. Divide the stew into bowls and serve.

95. Chicken And Cucumber Salad

Servings: 4
Cooking Time: 10 Minutes
Ingredients:
- 1 cucumber, chopped
- 1 tablespoon ricotta cheese
- 1 tablespoon mascarpone cheese
- ½ cup Monterey Jack cheese, grated
- 1-pound chicken breast, skinless, boneless
- 1 teaspoon avocado oil
- ½ teaspoon salt
- 1 teaspoon dried oregano
- 1 teaspoon ground black pepper
- 1 teaspoon ground paprika
- 1 oz bacon, chopped

Directions:
1. Rub the chicken breast with salt, dried oregano, ground black pepper, and ground paprika. Then put the chopped bacon in the air fryer basket. Place the chicken breast over the bacon and sprinkle with avocado oil. Cook the ingredients for 10 minutes at 395F. Meanwhile, in the shallow bowl mix up mascarpone cheese and ricotta cheese. Put the chopped cucumber in the salad bowl. Add grated Monterey jack cheese. When the chicken and bacon are cooked, remove them from the air fryer basket. Chop the chicken breast into tiny pieces and add in the salad bowl Add bacon and mascarpone mixture. Stir the salad with the help of the spatula.

96. Pepperoni Pizza

Servings: 3

Cooking Time: 15 Minutes
Ingredients:
- 3 portobello mushroom caps, cleaned and scooped
- 3 tbsp. olive oil
- 3 tbsp. tomato sauce
- 3 tbsp. mozzarella, shredded
- 12 slices pepperoni
- 1 pinch salt
- 1 pinch dried Italian seasonings

Directions:
1. Pre-heat the Air Fryer to 330°F.
2. Season both sides of the portobello mushrooms with a drizzle of olive oil, then sprinkle salt and the Italian seasonings on the insides.
3. With a knife, spread the tomato sauce evenly over the mushroom, before adding the mozzarella on top.
4. Put the portobello in the cooking basket and place in the Air Fryer.
5. Cook for 1 minute, before taking the cooking basket out of the fryer and putting the pepperoni slices on top.
6. Cook for another 3 to 5 minutes. Garnish with freshly grated parmesan cheese and crushed red pepper flakes and serve.

97. Chicken And Arugula Salad

Servings: 2
Cooking Time: 12 Minutes
Ingredients:
- 2 bacon slices, cooked, chopped
- 2 cups arugula, chopped
- 10 oz chicken breast, skinless, boneless
- 1 teaspoon ground black pepper
- ½ teaspoon salt
- 1 teaspoon avocado oil
- ½ teaspoon ground cumin
- ½ teaspoon ground paprika
- 1 tablespoon olive oil
- ¼ teaspoon minced garlic
- 1 teaspoon fresh cilantro, chopped

Directions:
1. Rub the chicken breast with ground black pepper, salt, ground cumin, ground paprika, and avocado oil. Then preheat the air fryer to 365F. Put the chicken breast in the preheated air fryer and cook for 12 minutes. Meanwhile, in the salad bowl mix up chopped bacon, arugula, and fresh cilantro. In the shallow bowl mix up minced garlic and olive oil. Chop the cooked chicken breasts and add in the salad mixture. Sprinkle the salad with garlic oil and shake well.

98. Mozzarella Bruschetta

Servings: 1

Cooking Time: 10 Minutes

Ingredients:
- 6 small loaf slices
- ½ cup tomatoes, finely chopped
- 3 oz. mozzarella cheese, grated
- 1 tbsp. fresh basil, chopped
- 1 tbsp. olive oil

Directions:
1. Pre-heat the Air Fryer to 350°F. Place the bread inside and cook for about 3 minutes.
2. Add the tomato, mozzarella, prosciutto, and a drizzle of olive oil on top.
3. Cook the bruschetta for an additional minute before serving.

99. Pesto Gnocchi

Servings: 4
Cooking Time: 30 Minutes

Ingredients:
- 1 package [16-oz.] shelf-stable gnocchi
- 1 medium-sized onion, chopped
- 3 cloves garlic, minced
- 1 jar [8 oz.] pesto
- ⅓ cup parmesan cheese, grated
- 1 tbsp. extra virgin olive oil
- Salt and black pepper to taste

Directions:
1. Pre-heat the Air Fryer to 340°F.
2. In a large bowl combine the onion, garlic, and gnocchi, and drizzle with the olive oil. Mix thoroughly.
3. Transfer the mixture to the fryer and cook for 15 – 20 minutes, stirring occasionally, making sure the gnocchi become lightly brown and crispy.
4. Add in the pesto and Parmesan cheese, and give everything a good stir before serving straightaway.

100.Fried Pickles

Servings: 4
Cooking Time: 30 Minutes

Ingredients:
- 14 dill pickles, sliced
- ¼ cup flour
- 1/8 tsp. baking powder
- Pinch of salt
- 2 tbsp. cornstarch + 3 tbsp. water
- 6 tbsp. bread crumbs
- ½ tsp. paprika
- Cooking spray

Directions:
1. Pre-heat your Air Fryer at 400°F.
2. Drain any excess moisture out of the dill pickles on a paper towel.
3. In a bowl, combine the flour, baking powder and salt.
4. Throw in the cornstarch and water mixture and combine well with a whisk.

5. Put the panko bread crumbs in a shallow dish along with the paprika. Mix thoroughly.
6. Dip the pickles in the flour batter, before coating in the bread crumbs. Spritz all the pickles with the cooking spray.
7. Transfer to the fryer and cook for 15 minutes, until a golden brown color is achieved.

101.Cauliflower Bites

Servings: 4
Cooking Time: 30 Minutes

Ingredients:
- 1 cup flour
- ⅓ cup desiccated coconut
- Salt and pepper to taste
- 1 flax egg [1 tbsp. flaxseed meal + 3 tbsp. water]
- 1 small cauliflower, cut into florets
- 1 tsp. mixed spice
- ½ tsp. mustard powder
- 2 tbsp. maple syrup
- 1 clove of garlic, minced
- 2 tbsp. soy sauce

Directions:
1. Pre-heat the Air Fryer to 400°F.
2. In a bowl, mix together the oats, flour, and desiccated coconut, sprinkling with some salt and pepper as desired.
3. In a separate bowl, season the flax egg with a pinch of salt.
4. Coat the cauliflower with mixed spice and mustard powder.
5. Dip the florets into the flax egg, then into the flour mixture. Cook for 15 minutes in the fryer.
6. In the meantime, place a saucepan over medium heat and add in the maple syrup, garlic, and soy sauce. Boil first, before reducing the heat to allow the sauce to thicken.
7. Remove the florets from the Air Fryer and transfer to the saucepan. Coat the florets in the sauce before returning to the fryer and allowing to cook for an additional 5 minutes.

102.Italian Sausages

Servings: 4
Cooking Time: 12 Minutes

Ingredients:
- 4 pork Italian sausages
- ½ cup keto tomato sauce
- 4 Mozzarella sticks
- 1 teaspoon butter, softened

Directions:
1. Make the cross-section in every sausage with the help of the knife. Then fill the cut with the Mozzarella stick. Brush the air fryer pan with butter. Put the stuffed

sausages in the pan and sprinkle them with tomato sauce. Preheat the air fryer to 375F. Place the pan with sausages in the air fryer and cook them for 12 minutes or until the sausages are golden brown.

103.Italian Style Eggplant Sandwich

Servings: 4
Cooking Time:26 Minutes
Ingredients:
- 1 eggplant; sliced
- 2 tsp. parsley; dried
- 1/2 cup breadcrumbs
- 1/2 tsp. Italian seasoning
- 1/2 tsp. garlic powder
- 1/2 tsp. onion powder
- 2 tbsp. milk
- 4 bread slices
- Cooking spray
- 1/2 cup mayonnaise
- 3/4 cup tomato sauce
- 2 cups mozzarella cheese; grated
- Salt and black pepper to the taste

Directions:
1. Season eggplant slices with salt and pepper, leave aside for 10 minutes and then pat dry them well.
2. In a bowl; mix parsley with breadcrumbs, Italian seasoning, onion and garlic powder, salt and black pepper and stir.
3. In another bowl; mix milk with mayo and whisk well.
4. Brush eggplant slices with mayo mix, dip them in breadcrumbs, place them in your air fryer's basket, spray with cooking oil and cook them at 400 °F, for 15 minutes; flipping them after 8 minutes.
5. Brush each bread slice with olive oil and arrange 2 on a working surface.
6. Add mozzarella and parmesan on each, add baked eggplant slices; spread tomato sauce and basil and top with the other bread slices, greased side down. Divide sandwiches on plates; cut them in halves and serve for lunch.

104.Mustard Chicken

Servings: 4
Cooking Time: 30 Minutes
Ingredients:
- 1 and ½ pounds chicken thighs, bone-in
- 2 tablespoons Dijon mustard
- A pinch of salt and black pepper
- Cooking spray

Directions:
1. In a bowl, mix the chicken thighs with all the other ingredients and toss. Put the chicken in your Air Fryer's basket and cook at 370 degrees F for 30 minutes shaking

halfway. Serve these chicken thighs for lunch.

105.Bacon Pancetta Casserole

Servings: 4
Cooking Time: 20 Minutes
Ingredients:
- 2 cups cauliflower, shredded
- 3 oz pancetta, chopped
- 2 oz bacon, chopped
- 1 cup Cheddar cheese, shredded
- ½ cup heavy cream
- 1 teaspoon salt
- 1 teaspoon cayenne pepper
- 1 teaspoon dried oregano

Directions:
1. Put bacon and pancetta in the air fryer and cook it for 10 minutes at 400F. Stir the ingredients every 3 minutes to avoid burning. Then mix up shredded cauliflower and cooked pancetta and bacon. Add salt and cayenne pepper. Mix up the mixture. Add the dried oregano. Line the air fryer pan with baking paper and put the cauliflower mixture inside. Top it with Cheddar cheese and sprinkle with heavy cream. Cook the casserole for 10 minutes at 365F.

106.Herbed Butter Beef Loin

Servings: 4
Cooking Time: 25 Minutes
Ingredients:
- 1 tbsp. butter, melted
- ¼ dried thyme
- 1 tsp. garlic salt
- ¼ tsp. dried parsley
- 1 lb. beef loin

Directions:
1. In a bowl, combine the melted butter, thyme, garlic salt, and parsley.
2. Cut the beef loin into slices and generously apply the seasoned butter using a brush.
3. Pre-heat your fryer at 400°F and place a rack inside.
4. Cook the beef for fifteen minutes.
5. Take care when removing it and serve hot.

107.Meatballs Sandwich Delight

Servings: 4
Cooking Time:32 Minutes
Ingredients:
- 3 baguettes; sliced more than halfway through
- 14 oz. beef; ground
- 1 tbsp. olive oil
- 1 tsp. thyme; dried
- 1 tsp. basil; dried
- 7 oz. tomato sauce

- 1 small onion; chopped
- 1 egg; whisked
- 1 tbsp. bread crumbs
- 2 tbsp. cheddar cheese; grated
- 1 tbsp. oregano; chopped
- Salt and black pepper to the taste

Directions:
1. In a bowl; combine meat with salt, pepper, onion, breadcrumbs, egg, cheese, oregano, thyme and basil; stir, shape medium meatballs and add them to your air fryer after you've greased it with the oil.
2. Cook them at 375 °F, for 12 minutes; flipping them halfway.
3. Add tomato sauce, cook meatballs for 10 minutes more and arrange them on sliced baguettes. Serve them right away.

108.Pesto Stuffed Bella Mushrooms

Servings: 6
Cooking Time: 25 Minutes
Ingredients:
- 1 cup basil
- ½ cup cashew nuts, soaked overnight
- ½ cup nutritional yeast
- 1 tbsp. lemon juice
- 2 cloves of garlic
- 1 tbsp. olive oil
- Salt to taste
- 1 lb. baby Bella mushroom, stems removed

Directions:
1. Pre-heat the Air Fryer at 400°F.
2. Prepare your pesto. In a food processor, blend together the basil, cashew nuts, nutritional yeast, lemon juice, garlic and olive oil to combine well. Sprinkle on salt as desired.
3. Turn the mushrooms cap-side down and spread the pesto on the underside of each cap.
4. Transfer to the fryer and cook for 15 minutes.

109.Meatballs

Servings: 6
Cooking Time: 30 Minutes
Ingredients:
- 1 lb ground beef (or ½ lb beef, ½ lb pork)
- ½ cup grated parmesan cheese
- 1 tbsp minced garlic (or paste)
- ½ cup mozzarella cheese
- 1 tsp freshly ground pepper

Directions:
1. Preheat your fryer to 400°F/200°C.
2. In a bowl, mix all the ingredients together.
3. Roll the meat mixture into 5 generous meatballs.
4. Bake inside your fryer at 170°F/80°C for about 18 minutes.

5. Serve with sauce!

110.Ribs

Servings: 4
Cooking Time: 60 Minutes
Ingredients:
- 1 lb. pork ribs
- 1 tbsp. barbecue dry rub
- 1 tsp. mustard
- 1 tbsp. apple cider vinegar
- 1 tsp. sesame oil

Directions:
1. Chop up the pork ribs.
2. Combine the dry rub, mustard, apple cider vinegar, and sesame oil, then coat the ribs with this mixture. Refrigerate the ribs for twenty minutes.
3. Preheat the fryer at 360°F.
4. When the ribs are ready, place them in the fryer and cook for 15 minutes. Flip them and cook on the other side for a further fifteen minutes. Then serve and enjoy!

111.Sage Chicken Escallops

Servings: 4
Cooking Time: 45 Minutes
Ingredients:
- 4 skinless chicken breasts
- 2 eggs, beaten
- ½ cup flour
- 6 sage leaves
- ¼ cup bread crumbs
- ¼ cup parmesan cheese
- Cooking spray

Directions:
1. Cut the chicken breasts into thin, flat slices.
2. In a bowl, combine the parmesan with the sage.
3. Add in the flour and eggs and sprinkle with salt and pepper as desired. Mix well.
4. Dip chicken in the flour-egg mixture.
5. Coat the chicken in the panko bread crumbs.
6. Spritz the inside of the Air Fryer with cooking spray and set it to 390°F, allowing it to warm.
7. Cook the chicken for 20 minutes.
8. When golden, serve with fried rice.

112.Steak And Cabbage

Servings: 4
Cooking Time:20 Minutes
Ingredients:
- 1/2 lb. sirloin steak; cut into strips
- 2 green onions; chopped.
- 2 garlic cloves; minced
- 2 tsp. cornstarch
- 1 tbsp. peanut oil
- 2 cups green cabbage; chopped
- 1 yellow bell pepper; chopped

- Salt and black pepper to the taste

Directions:
1. In a bowl; mix cabbage with salt, pepper and peanut oil; toss, transfer to air fryer's basket, cook at 370 °F, for 4 minutes and transfer to a bowl.
2. Add steak strips to your air fryer; also add green onions, bell pepper, garlic, salt and pepper, toss and cook for 5 minutes. Add over cabbage; toss, divide among plates and serve for lunch.

113.Cheeseburger Sliders

Servings: 3
Cooking Time: 20 Minutes
Ingredients:
- 1 lb. ground beef
- 6 slices cheddar cheese
- 6 dinner rolls
- Salt and pepper

Directions:
1. Pre-heat the Air Fryer to 390°F.
2. With your hands, shape the ground beef into 6 x 5-oz. patties. Sprinkle on some salt and pepper to taste.
3. Place the burgers in the cooking basket and cook for 10 minutes. Take care when removing them from the Air Fryer.
4. Top the patties with the cheese. Put them back in the Air Fryer and allow to cook for another minute before serving.

114.Pork And Zucchinis

Servings: 4
Cooking Time: 30 Minutes
Ingredients:
- 2 pounds pork stew meat, cubed
- 2 zucchinis, cubed
- Salt and black pepper to the taste
- ½ cup beef stock
- ½ teaspoon smoked paprika
- A handful cilantro, chopped

Directions:
1. In a pan that fits your air fryer, mix all the ingredients, toss, introduce in your air fryer and cook at 370 degrees F for 30 minutes. Divide into bowls and serve right away.

115.Sweet Potato Casserole

Servings: 6
Cooking Time:60 Minutes
Ingredients:
- 3 big sweet potatoes; pricked with a fork
- 1 cup chicken stock
- 1/4 tsp. nutmeg; ground
- 1/3 cup coconut cream
- Salt and black pepper to the taste
- A pinch of cayenne pepper

Directions:

1. Place sweet potatoes in your air fryer; cook them at 350 °F, for 40 minutes; cool them down, peel, roughly chop and transfer to a pan that fits your air fryer.
2. Add stock, salt, pepper, cayenne and coconut cream; toss, introduce in your air fryer and cook at 360 °F, for 10 minutes more. Divide casserole into bowls and serve.

116.Cheese Pizza

Servings: 4
Cooking Time: 15 Minutes
Ingredients:
- 1 pc. bread
- ½ lb. mozzarella cheese
- 1 tbsp. olive oil
- 2 tbsp. ketchup
- ⅓ cup sausage
- 1 tsp. garlic powder

Directions:
1. Using a tablespoon, spread the ketchup over the pita bread.
2. Top with the sausage and cheese. Season with the garlic powder and 1 tablespoon of olive oil.
3. Pre-heat the Air Fryer to 340°F.
4. Put the pizza in the fryer basket and cook for 6 minutes. Enjoy!

117.Baby Back Ribs

Servings: 2
Cooking Time: 45 Minutes
Ingredients:
- 2 tsp. red pepper flakes
- ¾ ground ginger
- 3 cloves minced garlic
- Salt and pepper
- 2 baby back ribs

Directions:
1. Pre-heat your fryer at 350°F.
2. Combine the red pepper flakes, ginger, garlic, salt and pepper in a bowl, making sure to mix well. Massage the mixture into the baby back ribs.
3. Cook the ribs in the fryer for thirty minutes.
4. Take care when taking the rubs out of the fryer. Place them on a serving dish and enjoy with a low-carb barbecue sauce of your choosing.

118.Pulled Pork

Servings: 1
Cooking Time: 30 Minutes
Ingredients:
- 1 lb. pork tenderloin
- 2 tbsp. barbecue dry rub
- 1/3 cup heavy cream
- 1 tsp. butter

Directions:

1. Pre-heat your fryer at 370°F.
2. Massage the dry rub of your choice into the tenderloin, coating it well.
3. Cook the tenderloin in the fryer for twenty minutes. When cooked, shred with two forks.
4. Add the heavy cream and butter into the fryer along with the shredded pork and stir well. Cook for a further four minutes.
5. Allow to cool a little, then serve and enjoy.

119.Veggie Pizza

Servings: 4
Cooking Time: 15 Minutes
Ingredients:
- 8 bacon slices
- ¼ cup black olives, sliced
- ¼ cup scallions, sliced
- 1 green bell pepper, sliced
- 1 cup Mozzarella, shredded
- 1 tablespoon keto tomato sauce
- ½ teaspoon dried basil
- ½ teaspoon sesame oil

Directions:
1. Line the air fryer pan with baking paper. Then make the layer of the sliced bacon in the pan and sprinkle gently with sesame oil. Preheat the air fryer to 400F. Place the pan with the bacon in the air fryer basket and cook it for 9 minutes at 400F. After this, sprinkle the bacon with keto tomato sauce and top with Mozzarella. Then add bell pepper, spring onions, and black olives. Sprinkle the pizza with dried basil and cook for 6 minutes at 400F.

120.Pork And Eggs Bowls

Servings: 4
Cooking Time: 15 Minutes
Ingredients:
- 2 eggs, whisked
- 1 and ½ pounds pork meat, ground
- 2 teaspoons olive oil
- ½ cup keto tomato sauce

- Salt and black pepper to the taste

Directions:
1. Heat up a pan that fits the Air Fryer with the oil over medium-high heat, add the meat and brown for 3-4 minutes. Add the rest of the ingredients, toss, put the pan in the machine and cook at 370 degrees F for 12 minutes. Divide into bowls and serve for lunch with a side salad.

121.Pork And Okra Stew

Servings: 4
Cooking Time: 20 Minutes
Ingredients:
- 1 and ½ pounds pork stew meat, cubed and browned
- 2 teaspoons sweet paprika
- 1 tablespoon olive oil
- 1 cup okra
- Salt and black pepper to the taste
- 3 garlic cloves, minced

Directions:
1. In your air fryer's pan, combine the meat with the remaining ingredients, toss, cover and cook at 370 degrees F for 20 minutes. Divide the stew into bowls and serve.

122.Beef And Sauce

Servings: 4
Cooking Time: 20 Minutes
Ingredients:
- 1 pound lean beef meat, cubed and browned
- 2 garlic cloves, minced
- Salt and black pepper to the taste
- Cooking spray
- 16 ounces keto tomato sauce

Directions:
1. Preheat the Air Fryer at 400 degrees F, add the pan inside, grease it with cooking spray, add the meat and all the other ingredients, toss and cook for 20 minutes. Divide into bowls and serve for lunch.

VEGETABLE & SIDE DISHES

123.Fried Peppers With Sriracha Mayo

Servings: 2
Cooking Time: 20 Minutes
Ingredients:
- 4 bell peppers, seeded and sliced (1-inch pieces)
- 1 onion, sliced (1-inch pieces)
- 1 tablespoon olive oil
- 1/2 teaspoon dried rosemary
- 1/2 teaspoon dried basil
- Kosher salt, to taste
- 1/4 teaspoon ground black pepper
- 1/3 cup mayonnaise
- 1/3 teaspoon Sriracha

Directions:
1. Toss the bell peppers and onions with the olive oil, rosemary, basil, salt, and black pepper.
2. Place the peppers and onions on an even layer in the cooking basket. Cook at 400 degrees F for 12 to 14 minutes.
3. Meanwhile, make the sauce by whisking the mayonnaise and Sriracha. Serve immediately.

124.Coconut Risotto

Servings: 4
Cooking Time: 20 Minutes
Ingredients:
- 2 cups cauliflower rice
- 1 cup coconut milk
- 2 tablespoons coconut oil, melted
- 1 tablespoon cilantro, chopped
- 1 tablespoon olive oil
- 1 teaspoon lime zest, grated
- 2 tablespoons parmesan, grated

Directions:
1. In a pan that fits your air fryer, mix all the ingredients, stir, introduce in the fryer and cook at 360 degrees F for 20 minutes. Divide between plates and serve as a side dish.

125.Pumpkin Wedges

Servings:3
Cooking Time: 30 Minutes
Ingredients:
- 1 tbsp paprika
- 1 whole lime, squeezed
- 1 cup paleo dressing
- 1 tbsp balsamic vinegar
- Salt and pepper to taste
- 1 tsp turmeric

Directions:
1. Preheat your air fryer to 360 F. Add the pumpkin wedges in your air fryer's cooking basket, and cook for 20 minutes. In a mixing bowl, mix lime juice, vinegar, turmeric, salt, pepper and paprika to form a marinade. Pour the marinade over pumpkin, and cook for 5 more minutes.

126.Chili Cheese Balls

Servings:6
Cooking Time: 20 Minutes
Ingredients:
- 2 cups grated Parmesan cheese
- 2 red potatoes, boiled and mashed
- 1 medium onion, finely chopped
- 1 ½ tsp red chili flakes
- 1 green chili, finely chopped
- Salt to taste
- 4 tbsp chopped cilantro
- 1 cup flour
- 1 cup breadcrumbs

Directions:
1. In a bowl, combine cottage cheese, Parmesan, onion, chili flakes, green chili, salt, cilantro, flour, and mash. Mold out balls and roll in breadcrumbs. Put in the fryer basket and cook for 15 minutes at 350 F.

127.Balsamic Potatoes Recipe

Servings: 4
Cooking Time:30 Minutes
Ingredients:
- 1 ½ lbs. baby potatoes; halved
- 2 garlic cloves; chopped.
- 2 red onions; chopped
- 1 ½ tbsp. balsamic vinegar
- 2 thyme springs; chopped
- 9 oz. cherry tomatoes
- 3 tbsp. olive oil
- Salt and black pepper to the taste

Directions:
1. In your food processor, mix garlic with onions, oil, vinegar, thyme, salt and pepper and pulse really well.
2. In a bowl; mix potatoes with tomatoes and balsamic marinade, toss well, transfer to your air fryer and cook at 380 °F, for 20 minutes. Divide among plates and serve

128.Spicy Cabbage

Servings: 4
Cooking Time: 12 Minutes
Ingredients:
- 1 green cabbage head, shredded
- 1 tablespoon olive oil
- 1 teaspoon cayenne pepper
- A pinch of salt and black pepper
- 2 teaspoons sweet paprika

Directions:

1. Mix all of the ingredients in a pan that fits your fryer.
2. Place the pan in the fryer and cook at 320 degrees F for 12 minutes.
3. Divide between plates and serve right away.

129.Cheesy Zucchini Tots

Servings: 4
Cooking Time: 6 Minutes
Ingredients:
- 1 zucchini, grated
- ½ cup Mozzarella, shredded
- 1 egg, beaten
- 2 tablespoons almond flour
- ½ teaspoon ground black pepper
- 1 teaspoon coconut oil, melted

Directions:
1. Mix up grated zucchini, shredded Mozzarella, egg, almond flour, and ground black pepper. Then make the small zucchini tots with the help of the fingertips. Preheat the air fryer to 385F. Place the zucchini tots in the air fryer basket and cook for 3 minutes from each side or until the zucchini tots are golden brown.

130.Plums & Pancetta Bombs

Servings:10
Cooking Time: 25 Minutes
Ingredients:
- 2 tbsp fresh rosemary, finely chopped
- 1 cup almonds, chopped into small pieces
- Salt and black pepper
- 15 dried plums, chopped
- 15 pancetta slices

Directions:
1. Line the air fryer basket with baking paper. In a bowl, add cheese, rosemary, almonds, salt, pepper and plums; stir well. Roll into balls and wrap with a pancetta slice. Arrange the bombs on the fryer and cook for 10 minutes at 400 F. Let cool before removing them from the air fryer. Serve with toothpicks.

131.Spanish-style Eggs With Manchego Cheese

Servings: 4
Cooking Time: 40 Minutes
Ingredients:
- 1/3 cup grated Manchego, cheese
- 5 eggs
- 1 small onion, finely chopped
- 2 green garlic stalks, peeled and finely minced
- 1 ½ cups white mushrooms, chopped
- 1 teaspoon dried basil
- 1 ½ tablespoons olive oil
- 3/4 teaspoon dried oregano
- 1/2 teaspoon dried parsley flakes or 1 tablespoon fresh flat-leaf Italian parsley
- 1 teaspoon porcini powder
- Table salt and freshly ground black pepper, to savor

Directions:
1. Start by preheating your Air Fryer to 350 degrees F. Add the oil, mushrooms, onion, and green garlic to the Air Fryer baking dish. Bake this mixture for 6 minutes or until it is tender.
2. Meanwhile, crack the eggs into a mixing bowl; beat the eggs until they're well whisked. Next, add the seasonings and mix again. Pause your Air Fryer and take the baking dish out of the basket.
3. Pour the whisked egg mixture into the baking dish with sautéed mixture. Top with the grated Manchego cheese.
4. Bake for about 32 minutes at 320 degrees F or until your frittata is set. Serve warm. Bon appétit!

132.Garlic Lemony Asparagus

Servings: 4
Cooking Time: 15 Minutes
Ingredients:
- 1 bunch asparagus, trimmed
- Salt and black pepper to the taste
- 4 tablespoons olive oil
- 4 garlic cloves, minced
- Juice of ½ lemon
- 3 tablespoons parmesan, grated

Directions:
1. In a bowl, mix the asparagus with all the ingredients except the parmesan, toss, transfer it to your air fryer's basket and cook at 400 degrees F for 15 minutes. Divide between plates, sprinkle the parmesan on top and serve as a side dish.

133.Mozzarella Green Beans

Servings: 4
Cooking Time: 6 Minutes
Ingredients:
- 1 cup green beans, trimmed
- 2 oz Mozzarella, shredded
- 1 teaspoon butter
- ½ teaspoon chili flakes
- ¼ cup beef broth

Directions:
1. Sprinkle the green beans with chili flakes and put in the air fryer baking pan. Add beef broth and butter. Then top the vegetables with shredded Mozzarella. Preheat the air fryer to 400F. Put the pan with green beans in the air fryer and cook the meal for 6 minutes.

134.Easy Veggie Fried Balls

Servings: 3
Cooking Time: 30 Minutes
Ingredients:
- 1/2 pound sweet potatoes, grated
- 1 cup carrots
- 1 cup corn
- 2 garlic cloves, minced
- 1 shallot, chopped
- Sea salt and ground black pepper, to taste
- 2 tablespoons fresh parsley, chopped
- 1 egg, well beaten
- 1/2 cup purpose flour
- 1/2 cup Romano cheese, grated
- 1/2 cup dried bread flakes
- 1 tablespoon olive oil

Directions:
1. Mix the veggies, spices, egg, flour, and Romano cheese until everything is well incorporated.
2. Take 1 tablespoon of the veggie mixture and roll into a ball. Roll the balls onto the dried bread flakes. Brush the veggie balls with olive oil on all sides.
3. Cook in the preheated Air Fryer at 360 degrees F for 15 minutes or until thoroughly cooked and crispy.
4. Repeat the process until you run out of ingredients. Bon appétit!

135.Cayenne Pepper Wings With Gorgonzola Dip

Servings:4
Cooking Time: 30 Minutes
Ingredients:
- 1 tsp cayenne pepper
- Salt to taste
- 2 tbsp grapeseed oil
- 2 tsp chili flakes
- 1 cup heavy cream
- 3 oz gorgonzola cheese, crumbled
- ½ lemon, juiced
- ½ tsp garlic powder

Directions:
1. Preheat air fryer to 380 F. Coat the chicken with cayenne pepper, salt, and oil. Place in the basket and cook for 20 minutes. In a bowl, mix heavy cream, gorgonzola cheese, lemon juice, and garlic powder.Serve with chicken wings.

136.Sweet Corn Fritters With Avocado

Servings: 3
Cooking Time: 20 Minutes
Ingredients:
- 2 cups sweet corn kernels
- 1 small-sized onion, chopped
- 1 garlic clove, minced
- 2 eggs, whisked
- 1 teaspoon baking powder
- 2 tablespoons fresh cilantro, chopped
- Sea salt and ground black pepper, to taste
- 1 avocado, peeled, pitted and diced
- 2 tablespoons sweet chili sauce

Directions:
1. In a mixing bowl, thoroughly combine the corn, onion, garlic, eggs, baking powder, cilantro, salt, and black pepper.
2. Shape the corn mixture into 6 patties and transfer them to the lightly greased Air Fryer basket.
3. Cook in the preheated Air Fry at 370 degrees for 8 minutes; turn them over and cook for 7 minutes longer.
4. Serve the fritters with the avocado and chili sauce.

137.Baked Cauliflower

Servings: 2
Cooking Time: 35 Minutes
Ingredients:
- 1/2 cauliflower head, cut into florets
- 2 tbsp olive oil
- For seasoning:
- 1/2 tsp ground cumin
- 1/2 tsp black pepper
- 1/2 tsp white pepper
- 1 tsp onion powder
- 1 tbsp ground cayenne pepper
- 1/4 tsp dried oregano
- 1/4 tsp dried basil
- 1/4 tsp dried thyme
- 1/2 tsp garlic powder
- 2 tbsp ground paprika
- 2 tsp salt

Directions:
1. Preheat the air fryer to 370 F.
2. In a large bowl, mix together all seasoning ingredients. Add oil and stir well.
3. Add cauliflower to the bowl seasoning mixture and stir to coat.
4. Transfer cauliflower florets into the air fryer basket and cook for 30-35 minutes. Shake basket 3-4 times while cooking.
5. Serve and enjoy.

138.Spiced Almonds

Servings:4
Cooking Time: 15 Minutes
Ingredients:
- ½ tsp smoked paprika
- 1 cup almonds
- 1 egg white
- Sea salt to taste

Directions:
1. Preheat the Air fryer to 310 F. Grease the air fryer basket with cooking spray. In a

bowl, whisk the egg white with cinnamon and paprika. Stir in almonds. Spread the almonds on the bottom of the air fryer basket and cook for 12 minutes, shaking once. Sprinkle with sea salt to serve.

139.Low-carb Pizza Crust

Servings: 4
Cooking Time: 20 Minutes
Ingredients:
- 1 tbsp. full-fat cream cheese
- ½ cup whole-milk mozzarella cheese, shredded
- 2 tbsp. flour
- 1 egg white

Directions:
1. In a microwave-safe bowl, combine the cream cheese, mozzarella, and flour and heat in the microwave for half a minute. Mix well to create a smooth consistency. Add in the egg white and stir to form a soft ball of dough.
2. With slightly wet hands, press the dough into a pizza crust about six inches in diameter.
3. Place a sheet of parchment paper in the bottom of your fryer and lay the crust on top. Cook for ten minutes at 350°F, turning the crust over halfway through the cooking time.
4. Top the pizza base with the toppings of your choice and enjoy!

140.Thyme & Garlic Sweet Potato Wedges

Servings:2
Cooking Time: 30 Minutes
Ingredients:
- 1 tbsp olive oil
- ¼ tsp salt
- ½ tsp chili powder
- ½ tsp garlic powder
- ½ tsp smoked paprika
- ½ tsp dried thyme
- A pinch cayenne pepper

Directions:
1. In a bowl, mix olive oil, salt, chili and garlic powder, smoked paprika, thyme, and cayenne. Toss in the potato wedges. Arrange the wedges on the air fryer, and cook for 25 minutes at 380 F, flipping once.

141.Basil Tomato And Eggplant Mix

Servings: 2
Cooking Time: 15 Minutes
Ingredients:
- 1 large eggplant
- 1 tablespoon keto tomatoes sauce
- 2 oz Mozzarella, sliced
- 1 tablespoon fresh basil

- ½ tomato, sliced
- 1 teaspoon olive oil
- ½ teaspoon ground black pepper

Directions:
1. Trim the eggplant from one side and cut it in the shape of Hasselback. Then sprinkle it with ground black pepper and olive oil. After this, fill the eggplant Hasselback with sliced Mozzarella, basil, and tomato one-by-one. Preheat the air fryer to 400F. Brush the eggplant with marinara sauce and place it in the air fryer. Cook the vegetable for 15 minutes. Cool the cooked eggplant to the room temperature and transfer in the serving plates.

142.Famous Fried Pickles

Servings: 6
Cooking Time: 20 Minutes
Ingredients:
- 1/3 cup milk
- 1 teaspoon garlic powder
- 2 medium-sized eggs
- 1 teaspoon fine sea salt
- 1/3 teaspoon chili powder
- 1/3 cup all-purpose flour
- 1/2 teaspoon shallot powder
- 2 jars sweet and sour pickle spears

Directions:
1. Pat the pickle spears dry with a kitchen towel. Then, take two mixing bowls.
2. Whisk the egg and milk in a bowl. In another bowl, combine all dry ingredients.
3. Firstly, dip the pickle spears into the dry mix; then coat each pickle with the egg/milk mixture; dredge them in the flour mixture again for additional coating.
4. Air fry battered pickles for 15 minutes at 385 degrees. Enjoy!

143.Cumin Artichokes

Servings: 4
Cooking Time: 15 Minutes
Ingredients:
- 12 ounces artichoke hearts
- ½ teaspoon olive oil
- 1 teaspoon coriander, ground
- ½ teaspoon cumin seeds
- Salt and black pepper to the taste
- 1 tablespoon lemon juice

Directions:
1. In a pan that fits your air fryer, mix all the ingredients, toss, introduce the pan in the fryer and cook at 370 degrees F for 15 minutes. Divide the mix between plates and serve as a side dish.

144.Bacon Green Beans Mix

Servings: 4

Cooking Time: 13 Minutes
Ingredients:
- 1 cup green beans, trimmed
- 4 oz bacon, sliced
- ¼ teaspoon salt
- 1 tablespoon avocado oil

Directions:
1. Wrap the green beans in the sliced bacon. After this, sprinkle the vegetables with salt and avocado oil. Preheat the air fryer to 385F. Carefully arrange the green beans in the air fryer in one layer and cook them for 5 minutes. Then flip the green beans on another side and cook for 8 minutes more.

145.Avocado And Green Beans

Servings: 4
Cooking Time: 15 Minutes
Ingredients:
- 1 pint mixed cherry tomatoes, halved
- 1 avocado, peeled, pitted and cubed
- ¼ pound green beans, trimmed and halved
- 2 tablespoons olive oil

Directions:
1. In a pan that fits your air fryer, mix the tomatoes with the rest of the ingredients, toss, put the pan in the machine and cook at 360 degrees F for 15 minutes. Transfer to bowls and serve.

146.Lemongrass Rice Mix

Servings: 4
Cooking Time: 10 Minutes
Ingredients:
- ½ cup broccoli, shredded
- ½ cup cauliflower, shredded
- ¼ teaspoon lemongrass
- 1 teaspoon ground turmeric
- ¼ cup beef broth
- 1 teaspoon butter
- ½ teaspoon salt
- 3 oz Cheddar cheese, shredded

Directions:
1. In the mixing bowl mix up shredded broccoli and cauliflower. Add lemongrass, turmeric, and salt. Then transfer the mixture in the air fryer baking pan and add beef broth. Add butter and top the keto rice with Cheddar cheese. Preheat the air fryer to 365F. Put the pan with "rice" in the air fryer and cook it for 10 minutes.

147.Mushroom Tots

Servings: 2
Cooking Time: 6 Minutes
Ingredients:
- 1 cup white mushrooms, grinded
- 1 teaspoon onion powder
- 1 egg yolk
- 3 teaspoons flax meal
- ½ teaspoon ground black pepper
- 1 teaspoon avocado oil
- 1 tablespoon coconut flour

Directions:
1. Mix up grinded white mushrooms with onion powder, egg yolk, flax meal, ground black pepper, and coconut flour. When the mixture is smooth and homogenous, make the mushroom tots. Preheat the air fryer to 400F. Sprinkle the air fryer basket with melted coconut oil and put the mushroom tots inside. Cook them for 3 minutes. Then flip the mushroom tots on another side and cook them for 2-3 minutes more or until they are light brown.

148.Basic Pepper French Fries

Servings:4
Cooking Time:33 Minutes
Ingredients:
- 1 teaspoon fine sea salt
- 1/2 teaspoon freshly ground black pepper
- 2 ½ tablespoons canola oil
- 6 Russet potatoes, cut them into fries
- 1/2 teaspoon crushed red pepper flakes

Directions:
1. Start by preheating your air fryer to 340 degrees F.
2. Place the fries in your air fryer and toss them with the oil. Add the seasonings and toss again.
3. Cook for 30 minutes, shaking your fries several times. Taste for doneness and eat warm.

149.Jalapeno Clouds

Servings: 4
Cooking Time: 4 Minutes
Ingredients:
- 2 egg whites
- 1 jalapeno pepper
- 1 teaspoon almond flour
- 1 oz Jarlsberg cheese, grated

Directions:
1. Whisk the egg whites until you get the strong peaks. After this, carefully mix up egg white peaks, almond flour, and Jarlsberg cheese. Slice the jalapeno pepper on 4 slices. Preheat the air fryer to 385F. Line the air fryer basket with baking paper. With the help of the spoon make the egg white clouds on the baking paper. Top the clouds with sliced jalapeno. Cook them for 4 minutes or until the clouds are light brown.

150.Ghee Lemony Endives

Servings: 4
Cooking Time: 15 Minutes

Ingredients:
- 3 tablespoons ghee, melted
- 12 endives, trimmed
- A pinch of salt and black pepper
- 1 tablespoon lemon juice

Directions:
1. In a bowl, mix the endives with the ghee, salt, pepper and lemon juice and toss. Put the endives in the fryer's basket and cook at 350 degrees F for 15 minutes. Divide between plates and serve.

151.Dill Green Beans

Servings: 4
Cooking Time: 15 Minutes
Ingredients:
- 1 pound green beans, trimmed
- 1 tablespoon coconut oil, melted
- 2 garlic cloves, minced
- Salt and black pepper to the taste
- ½ cup bacon, cooked and chopped
- 2 tablespoons dill, chopped

Directions:
1. In a pan that fits the air fryer, combine the green beans with the rest of the ingredients, toss, put the pan in the machine and cook at 390 degrees F for 15 minutes. Divide everything between plates and serve.

152.Summer Vegetable Fritters

Servings: 2
Cooking Time: 20 Minutes
Ingredients:
- 1 zucchini, grated and squeezed
- 1 cup cauliflower florets, boiled
- 4 tablespoons Romano cheese, grated
- 2 tablespoons fresh shallots, minced
- 1 teaspoon fresh garlic, minced
- 1 tablespoon peanut oil
- Sea salt and ground black pepper, to taste
- 1 teaspoon cayenne pepper

Directions:
1. In a mixing bowl, thoroughly combine all ingredients until everything is well incorporated.
2. Shape the mixture into patties. Spritz the Air Fryer basket with cooking spray.
3. Cook in the preheated Air Fryer at 365 degrees F for 6 minutes. Turn them over and cook for a further 6 minutes
4. Serve immediately and enjoy!

153.Japanese Tempura Bowl

Servings: 3
Cooking Time: 20 Minutes
Ingredients:
- 1 cup all-purpose flour
- Kosher salt and ground black pepper, to taste

- 1/2 teaspoon paprika
- 2 eggs
- 3 tablespoons soda water
- 1 cup panko crumbs
- 2 tablespoons olive oil
- 1 cup green beans
- 1 onion, cut into rings
- 1 zucchini, cut into slices
- 2 tablespoons soy sauce
- 1 tablespoon mirin
- 1 teaspoon dashi granules

Directions:
1. In a shallow bowl, mix the flour, salt, black pepper, and paprika. In a separate bowl, whisk the eggs and soda water. In a third shallow bowl, combine the panko crumbs with olive oil.
2. Dip the vegetables in flour mixture, then in the egg mixture; lastly, roll over the panko mixture to coat evenly.
3. Cook in the preheated Air Fryer at 400 degrees F for 10 minutes, shaking the basket halfway through the cooking time. Work in batches until the vegetables are crispy and golden brown.
4. Then, make the sauce by whisking the soy sauce, mirin, and dashi granules. Bon appétit!

154.Rosemary Green Beans

Servings: 1
Cooking Time: 10 Minutes
Ingredients:
- 1 tbsp. butter, melted
- 2 tbsp. rosemary
- ½ tsp. salt
- 3 cloves garlic, minced
- ¾ cup green beans, chopped

Directions:
1. Pre-heat your fryer at 390°F.
2. Combine the melted butter with the rosemary, salt, and minced garlic. Toss in the green beans, making sure to coat them well.
3. Cook in the fryer for five minutes.

155.Cheesy Sticks With Sweet Thai Sauce

Servings:4
Cooking Time: 20 Minutes + Freezing Time
Ingredients:
- 2 cups breadcrumbs
- 3 eggs
- 1 cup sweet Thai sauce
- 4 tbsp skimmed milk

Directions:
1. Pour crumbs in a bowl. Beat eggs into another bowl with milk. One after the other, dip sticks in the egg mixture, in the crumbs,

then egg mixture again and then in the crumbs again. Freeze for 1 hour.
2. Preheat air fryer to 380 F. Arrange the sticks on the fryer. Cook for 5 minutes, flipping them halfway through cooking to brown evenly. Cook in batches. Serve with a sweet Thai sauce.

156.Creamy Cauliflower And Broccoli

Servings: 6
Cooking Time: 20 Minutes
Ingredients:
- 1 pound cauliflower florets
- 1 pound broccoli florets
- 2 ½ tablespoons sesame oil
- 1/2 teaspoon smoked cayenne pepper
- 3/4 teaspoon sea salt flakes
- 1 tablespoon lemon zest, grated
- 1/2 cup Colby cheese, shredded

Directions:
1. Prepare the cauliflower and broccoli using your favorite steaming method. Then, drain them well; add the sesame oil, cayenne pepper, and salt flakes.
2. Air-fry at 390 degrees F for approximately 16 minutes; make sure to check the vegetables halfway through the cooking time.
3. Afterwards, stir in the lemon zest and Colby cheese; toss to coat well and serve immediately!

157.Air-fried Chickpeas With Herbs

Servings:4
Cooking Time: 20 Minutes
Ingredients:
- 2 tbsp olive oil
- 1 tsp dried rosemary
- ½ tsp dried thyme
- ¼ tsp dried sage
- ¼ tsp salt

Directions:
1. In a bowl, mix together chickpeas, oil, rosemary, thyme, sage, and salt. Transfer them to the air fryer and spread in an even layer. Cook 14 minutes at 380 F, shaking once, halfway through cooking.

158.Ghee Savoy Cabbage

Servings: 4
Cooking Time: 15 Minutes
Ingredients:
- 1 Savoy cabbage head, shredded
- Salt and black pepper to the taste
- 1 and ½ tablespoons ghee, melted
- ¼ cup coconut cream
- 1 tablespoon dill, chopped

Directions:

1. In a pan that fits the air fryer, combine all the ingredients except the coconut cream, toss, put the pan in the air fryer and cook at 390 degrees F for 10 minutes. Add the cream, toss, cook for 5 minutes more, divide between plates and serve.

159.Lemon Asparagus

Servings: 4
Cooking Time: 12 Minutes
Ingredients:
- 1 pound asparagus, trimmed
- A pinch of salt and black pepper
- 2 tablespoons olive oil
- 3 garlic cloves, minced
- 3 tablespoons parmesan, grated
- Juice of 1 lemon

Directions:
1. In a bowl, mix the asparagus with the rest of the ingredients and toss. Put the asparagus in your air fryer's basket and cook at 390 degrees F for 12 minutes. Divide between plates and serve.

160.Simple Cheese Sandwich

Servings:1
Cooking Time: 20 Minutes
Ingredients:
- 2 scallions
- 2 tbsp butter
- 2 slices bread
- ¾ cup Cheddar cheese

Directions:
1. Preheat your air fryer to 360 F.
2. Lay the bread slices on a flat surface. On one slice, spread the exposed side with butter, followed by cheddar and scallions. On the other slice, spread butter and then sprinkle cheese.
3. Bring the buttered sides together to form sand. Place the sandwich in your air fryer's cooking basket and cook for 10 minutes. Serve with berry sauce.

161.Mint-butter Stuffed Mushrooms

Servings:3
Cooking Time:19 Minutes
Ingredients:
- 3 garlic cloves, minced
- 1 teaspoon ground black pepper, or more to taste
- 1/3 cup seasoned breadcrumbs
- 1½ tablespoons fresh mint, chopped
- 1 teaspoon salt, or more to taste
- 1½ tablespoons melted butter
- 14 medium-sized mushrooms, cleaned, stalks removed

Directions:

1. Mix all of the above ingredients, minus the mushrooms, in a mixing bowl to prepare the filling.
2. Then, stuff the mushrooms with the prepared filling.
3. Air-fry stuffed mushrooms at 375 degrees F for about 12 minutes. Taste for doneness and serve at room temperature as a vegetarian appetizer.

162.Air Fried Green Tomatoes

Servings:1
Cooking Time: 7 Minutes
Ingredients:
- ½ cup panko breadcrumbs
- 3 tablespoons cornstarch
- ½ teaspoon dried basil, ground
- ½ teaspoon dried oregano, ground
- ½ teaspoon granulated onion
- Salt and pepper, to taste
- 1 medium-sized green tomato, sliced
- ½ teaspoon cooking oil

Directions:
1. In a mixing bowl, combine the panko breadcrumbs, cornstarch, basil, oregano, onion, salt, and pepper.
2. Dredge the tomato slices in the breadcrumb mixture.
3. Brush with oil and arrange on the double layer rack.
4. Place the rack with the dredged tomato slices in the air fryer.
5. Close the lid and cook for 7 minutes at 350°F.

163.Tomato Artichokes Mix

Servings: 4
Cooking Time: 15 Minutes
Ingredients:
- 14 ounces artichoke hearts, drained
- 1 tablespoon olive oil
- 2 cups black olives, pitted
- 3 garlic cloves, minced
- ½ cup keto tomato sauce
- 1 teaspoon garlic powder

Directions:
1. In a pan that fits your air fryer, mix the olives with the artichokes and the other ingredients, toss, put the pan in the fryer and cook at 350 degrees F for 15 minutes. Divide the mix between plates and serve.

164.Crispy Pepperoni Pizza

Servings:2
Cooking Time: 25 Minutes
Ingredients:
- Cooking spray
- ⅓ cup tomato sauce
- ⅓ cup mozzarella cheese, shredded

- 8 pepperonis, sliced
- Flour, to dust

Directions:
1. On a floured surface, place dough and dust with flour. Stretch with hands into an air-fryer fitting shape. Spray the air fryer basket with cooking spray and arrange the pizza inside. Brush generously with sauce, leaving some space at the border. scatter with mozzarella and top with pepperonis. Cook for 15 minutes, or until crispy, at 340 F.

165.Appetizing Cod Fingers

Servings:3
Cooking Time: 25 Minutes
Ingredients:
- Salt and pepper to taste
- 1 tsp seafood seasoning
- 2 eggs, beaten
- 1 cup cornmeal
- 1 pound cod fillets, cut into fingers
- 2 tbsp milk
- 2 eggs, beaten
- 1 cup breadcrumbs

Directions:
1. Preheat air fryer to 400 F. In a bowl, mix eggs with milk. In a separate bowl, mix flour, cornmeal, and seafood seasoning. In another bowl, mix spices with the eggs. In a third bowl, pour the breadcrumbs.
2. Dip cod fingers in the seasoned flour mixture, followed by a dip in the egg mixture and finally, coat with breadcrumbs. Place the prepared fingers in your air fryer's cooking basket and cook for 10 minutes.

166.Broccoli With Almonds

Servings: 4
Cooking Time: 16 Minutes
Ingredients:
- 1 1/2 lbs broccoli, cut into florets
- 3 tbsp olive oil
- 1 tbsp lemon juice
- 1/4 cup cheese, grated
- 3 tbsp slivered almonds, toasted
- 2 garlic cloves, sliced
- 1/4 tsp pepper
- 1/4 tsp salt

Directions:
1. Preheat the air fryer to 400 F.
2. Spray air fryer basket with cooking spray.
3. Add broccoli, pepper, salt, garlic, and oil in a large bowl and toss well.
4. Spread broccoli into the air fryer basket and cook for 16 minutes. Shake basket halfway through.

5. Add lemon juice, grated cheese, and almonds over broccoli and toss well.
6. Serve and enjoy.

167.Simple Taro Fries

Servings: 2
Cooking Time: 20 Minutes
Ingredients:
- 8 small taro, peel and cut into fries shape
- 1 tbsp olive oil
- 1/2 tsp salt

Directions:
1. Add taro slice in a bowl and toss well with olive oil and salt.
2. Transfer taro slices into the air fryer basket.
3. Cook at 360 F for 20 minutes. Toss halfway through.
4. Serve and enjoy.

168.Parmesan Cherry Tomatoes

Servings: 4
Cooking Time: 15 Minutes
Ingredients:
- 1 tablespoon ghee, melted
- 2 cups cherry tomatoes, halved
- 3 tablespoons scallions, chopped
- 1 teaspoon lemon zest, grated
- 2 tablespoons parsley, chopped
- ¼ cup parmesan, grated

Directions:
1. In a pan that fits the air fryer, combine all the ingredients except the parmesan, and toss. Sprinkle the parmesan on top, introduce the pan in the machine and cook at 360 degrees F for 10 minutes. Divide between plates and serve.

169.Zucchini Parmesan Chips

Servings:3
Cooking Time: 15 Minutes
Ingredients:
- 1 cup breadcrumbs
- 2 eggs, beaten
- 1 cup grated Parmesan cheese
- Salt and pepper to taste
- 1 tsp smoked paprika

Directions:
1. In a bowl, add breadcrumbs, salt, pepper, cheese, and paprika. Mix well. Dip zucchini slices in eggs and then in the cheese mix while pressing to coat them well. Spray the coated slices with cooking spray and put the in the fryer basket. Cook at 350 F for 8 minutes. Serve with salt spicy dip.

170.Turmeric Dill Cabbage

Servings: 4
Cooking Time: 15 Minutes
Ingredients:
- 1 green cabbage head, shredded
- ¼ cup ghee, melted
- 2 teaspoons turmeric powder
- 1 tablespoon dill, chopped

Directions:
1. In a pan that fits your air fryer, mix the cabbage with the rest of the ingredients except the dill, toss, put the pan in the fryer and cook at 370 degrees F for 15 minutes. Divide everything between plates and serve with dill sprinkled on top.

171.Cauliflower Patties

Servings: 2
Cooking Time: 10 Minutes
Ingredients:
- ¼ cup cauliflower, shredded
- 1 egg yolk
- ½ teaspoon ground turmeric
- ¼ teaspoon onion powder
- ¼ teaspoon salt
- 2 oz Cheddar cheese, shredded
- ¼ teaspoon baking powder
- 1 teaspoon heavy cream
- 1 tablespoon coconut flakes
- Cooking spray

Directions:
1. Squeeze the shredded cauliflower and put it in the bowl. Add egg yolk, ground turmeric, onion powder, baking powder, salt, heavy cream, and coconut flakes. Then melt Cheddar cheese and add it in the cauliflower mixture. Stir the ingredients until you get the smooth mass. After this, make the medium size cauliflower patties. Preheat the air fryer to 365F. Spray the air fryer basket with cooking spray and put the patties inside. Cook them for 5 minutes from each side.

172.Easy Celery Root Mix

Servings: 4
Cooking Time: 15 Minutes
Ingredients:
- 2 cups celery root, roughly cubed
- A pinch of salt and black pepper
- ½ tablespoon butter, melted

Directions:
1. Put all of the ingredients in your air fryer and toss.
2. Cook at 350 degrees F for 15 minutes.
3. Divide between plates and serve.

173.Cheese Lings

Servings: 6
Cooking Time: 25 Minutes
Ingredients:
- 1 cup flour
- small cubes cheese, grated

- ¼ tsp. chili powder
- 1 tsp. butter
- Salt to taste
- 1 tsp. baking powder

Directions:
1. Combine all the ingredients to form a dough, along with a small amount water as necessary.
2. Divide the dough into equal portions and roll each one into a ball.
3. Pre-heat Air Fryer at 360°F.
4. Transfer the balls to the fryer and air fry for 5 minutes, stirring periodically.

174.Tasty Herb Tomatoes

Servings: 4
Cooking Time: 15 Minutes
Ingredients:
- 2 large tomatoes, halved
- 1 tbsp olive oil
- 1/2 tsp thyme, chopped
- 2 garlic cloves, minced
- Pepper
- Salt

Directions:
1. Add all ingredients into the bowl and toss well.
2. Transfer tomatoes into the air fryer basket and cook at 390 F for 15 minutes.
3. Serve and enjoy.

175.Artichokes And Tarragon Sauce Dish

Servings: 4
Cooking Time:28 Minutes
Ingredients:
- 4 artichokes; trimmed
- 2 tbsp. tarragon; chopped
- 2 tbsp. lemon juice
- 1 celery stalk; chopped.
- 1/2 cup olive oil
- 2 tbsp. chicken stock
- Lemon zest from 2 lemons; grated
- Salt to the taste

Directions:
1. In your food processor; mix tarragon, chicken stock, lemon zest, lemon juice, celery, salt and olive oil and pulse very well.
2. In a bowl; mix artichokes with tarragon and lemon sauce; toss well, transfer them to your air fryer's basket and cook at 380 °F, for 18 minutes.
3. Divide artichokes on plates; drizzle the rest of the sauce all over and serve as a side dish.

176.Crumbed Beans

Servings: 4
Cooking Time: 10 Minutes
Ingredients:
- ½ cup flour

- 1 tsp. smoky chipotle powder
- ½ tsp. ground black pepper
- 1 tsp. sea salt flakes
- 2 eggs, beaten
- ½ cup crushed saltines
- 10 oz. wax beans

Directions:
1. Combine the flour, chipotle powder, black pepper, and salt in a bowl. Put the eggs in a second bowl. Place the crushed saltines in a third bowl.
2. Wash the beans with cold water and discard any tough strings.
3. Coat the beans with the flour mixture before dipping them into the beaten egg. Lastly cover them with the crushed saltines.
4. Spritz the beans with a cooking spray.
5. Air-fry at 360°F for 4 minutes. Give the cooking basket a good shake and continue to cook for 3 minutes. Serve hot.

177.Cheesy Bacon Fries

Servings:4
Cooking Time: 25 Minutes
Ingredients:
- 5 slices bacon, chopped
- 2 tbsp vegetable oil
- 2½ cups Cheddar cheese, shredded
- 3 oz melted cream cheese
- Salt and pepper to taste
- ¼ cup scallions, chopped

Directions:
1. Preheat your air fryer to 400 F.
2. Add bacon to air fryer's basket and cook for 4, shaking once; set aside. Add in potatoes and drizzle oil on top to coat. Cook for 25 minutes, shaking the basket every 5 minutes. Season with salt and pepper.
3. In a bowl, mix cheddar cheese and cream cheese. Pour over the potatoes and cook for 5 more minutes at 340 F. Sprinkle chopped scallions on top and serve.

178.Garlic Tomatoes Recipe

Servings: 4
Cooking Time:25 Minutes
Ingredients:
- 4 garlic cloves; crushed
- 1 lb. mixed cherry tomatoes
- 3 thyme springs; chopped.
- 1/4 cup olive oil
- Salt and black pepper to the taste

Directions:
1. In a bowl; mix tomatoes with salt, black pepper, garlic, olive oil and thyme, toss to coat, introduce in your air fryer and cook at 360 °F, for 15 minutes. Divide tomatoes mix on plates and serve

179.Tasty Okra

Servings: 2
Cooking Time: 12 Minutes
Ingredients:
- 1/2 lb okra, ends trimmed and sliced
- 1 tsp olive oil
- 1/2 tsp mango powder
- 1/2 tsp chili powder
- 1/2 tsp ground coriander
- 1/2 tsp ground cumin
- 1/8 tsp pepper
- 1/4 tsp salt

Directions:
1. Preheat the air fryer to 350 F.
2. Add all ingredients into the large bowl and toss well.
3. Spray air fryer basket with cooking spray.
4. Transfer okra mixture into the air fryer basket and cook for 10 minutes. Shake basket halfway through.
5. Toss okra well and cook for 2 minutes more.
6. Serve and enjoy.

180.Bell Pepper And Lettuce Side Salad

Servings: 4
Cooking Time: 15 Minutes
Ingredients:
- 1 tablespoon lemon juice
- 1 red bell pepper
- 1 lettuce head, torn
- Salt and black pepper to taste
- 3 tablespoons yogurt
- 2 tablespoons olive oil

Directions:
1. In your air fryer, place the bell pepper along with the oil, salt, and pepper; air fry at 400 degrees F for 15 minutes.
2. Cool the bell pepper down, peel, cut it into strips and put it in a bowl.
3. Add lettuce, lemon juice, yogurt, salt, and pepper.
4. Toss well, and serve as a side dish.

181.Beet Wedges Dish

Servings: 4
Cooking Time:25 Minutes
Ingredients:
- 4 beets; washed, peeled and cut into large wedges
- 1 tbsp. olive oil
- 2 garlic cloves; minced
- 1 tsp. lemon juice
- Salt and black to the taste

Directions:
1. In a bowl; mix beets with oil, salt, pepper, garlic and lemon juice; toss well, transfer to your air fryer's basket and cook them at 400 °F, for 15 minutes. Divide beets wedges on plates and serve as a side dish.

182.Crispy Squash

Servings:4
Cooking Time: 25 Minutes
Ingredients:
- 1 tbsp olive oil
- ¼ tsp salt
- ¼ tsp black pepper
- ¼ tsp dried thyme
- 1 tbsp finely chopped fresh parsley

Directions:
1. In a bowl, add squash, oil, salt, pepper, and thyme, and toss until squash is well-coated. Place squash in the air fryer and cook for 14 minutes at 360 F. Sprinkle with chopped parsley and serve chilled.

183.Nutmeg Kale

Servings: 4
Cooking Time: 15 Minutes
Ingredients:
- 1 tablespoon butter, melted
- ½ cup almond milk
- Salt and black pepper to the taste
- 3 garlic cloves
- 10 cups kale, roughly chopped
- ¼ teaspoon nutmeg, ground
- 1/3 cup parmesan, grated
- ¼ cup walnuts, chopped

Directions:
1. In a pan that fits the air fryer, combine all the ingredients, toss, introduce the pan in the machine and cook at 360 degrees F for 15 minutes. Divide between plates and serve.

VEGAN & VEGETARIAN RECIPES

184.Caramelized Carrots

Servings:3
Cooking Time:15 Minutes
Ingredients:
- 1 small bag baby carrots
- ½ cup butter, melted
- ½ cup brown sugar

Directions:
1. Preheat the Air fryer to 400 °F and grease an Air fryer basket.
2. Mix the butter and brown sugar in a bowl.
3. Add the carrots and toss to coat well.
4. Arrange the carrots in the Air fryer basket and cook for about 15 minutes.
5. Dish out and serve warm.

185.Minty Eggplant And Zucchini Bites

Servings: 8
Cooking Time: 35 Minutes
Ingredients:
- 2 teaspoons fresh mint leaves, chopped
- 1 ½ teaspoons red pepper chili flakes
- 2 tablespoons melted butter
- 1 pound eggplant, peeled and cubed
- 1 pound zucchini, peeled and cubed
- 3 tablespoons olive oil

Directions:
1. Toss all of the above ingredients in a large-sized mixing dish.
2. Roast the eggplant and zucchini bites for 30 minutes at 325 degrees F in your Air Fryer, turning once or twice.
3. Serve with a homemade dipping sauce.

186.Vegetable Skewers With Asian-style Peanut Sauce

Servings: 4
Cooking Time: 30 Minutes
Ingredients:
- 2 bell peppers, diced into 1-inch pieces
- 4 pearl onions, halved
- 8 small button mushrooms, cleaned
- 2 tablespoons extra-virgin olive oil
- Sea salt and ground black pepper, to taste
- 1 teaspoon red pepper flakes, crushed
- 1 teaspoon dried rosemary, crushed
- 1/3 teaspoon granulated garlic
- Peanut Sauce:
- 2 tablespoons peanut butter
- 1 tablespoon balsamic vinegar
- 1 tablespoon soy sauce
- 1/2 teaspoon garlic salt

Directions:
1. Soak the wooden skewers in water for 15 minutes.
2. Thread the vegetables on skewers; drizzle the olive oil all over the vegetable skewers; sprinkle with spices.
3. Cook in the preheated Air Fryer at 400 degrees F for 13 minutes.
4. Meanwhile, in a small dish, whisk the peanut butter with the balsamic vinegar, soy sauce, and garlic salt. Serve your skewers with the peanut sauce on the side. Enjoy!

187.Tofu In Sweet & Sour Sauce

Servings: 3
Cooking Time: 25 Minutes
Ingredients:
- 2 tablespoons Shoyu sauce
- 16 ounces extra-firm tofu, drained, pressed and cubed
- 1/2 cup water
- 1/4 cup pineapple juice
- 2 garlic cloves, minced
- 1/2 teaspoon fresh ginger, grated
- 1 teaspoon cayenne pepper
- 1/4 teaspoon ground black pepper
- 1/2 teaspoon salt
- 1 teaspoon honey
- 1 tablespoon arrowroot powder

Directions:
1. Drizzle the Shoyu sauce all over the tofu cubes. Cook in the preheated Air Fryer at 380 degrees F for 6 minutes; shake the basket and cook for a further 5 minutes.
2. Meanwhile, cook the remaining ingredients in a heavy skillet over medium heat for 10 minutes, until the sauce has slightly thickened.
3. Stir the fried tofu into the sauce and continue cooking for 4 minutes more or until the tofu is thoroughly heated.
4. Serve warm and enjoy!

188.Grilled Eggplant With Cumin-paprika Spice

Servings:2
Cooking Time: 20 Minutes
Ingredients:
- 1 Chinese eggplant, sliced into 1-inch thick circles
- 1 medium bell pepper, cut into chunks
- 1 tablespoon coriander seeds
- 1 tablespoon olive oil
- 1 teaspoon cumin
- 1 teaspoon paprika
- 1 teaspoon salt
- 1 zucchini, sliced into 1-inch thick circles
- 3 garlic cloves

Directions:

1. In a food processor, process garlic, coriander, olive oil, cumin, paprika, and salt until creamy.
2. Thread bell pepper, eggplant, and zucchini in skewers. Brush with garlic creamy paste. Place on skewer rack in air fryer.
3. For 10 minutes, cook on 360 °F. Halfway through cooking time, turnover skewers. If needed, cook in batches.
4. Serve and enjoy.

189.Air-fried Falafel

Servings:6
Cooking Time: 25 Minutes
Ingredients:
- ½ cup chickpea flour
- 1 cup fresh parsley, chopped
- Juice of 1 lemon
- 4 garlic cloves, chopped
- 1 onion, chopped
- 2 tsp ground cumin
- 2 tsp ground coriander
- 1 tsp chili powder
- Salt and black pepper

Directions:
1. In a blender, add chickpeas, flour, parsley, lemon juice, garlic, onion, cumin, coriander, chili, turmeric, salt and pepper, and blend until well-combined but not too battery; there should be some lumps. Shape the mixture into 15 balls and press them with hands, making sure they are still around.
2. Spray with oil and arrange them in a paper-lined air fryer basket; work in batches if needed. Cook at 360 F for 14 minutes, turning once halfway through. They should be crunchy and golden.

190.Simply Awesome Vegetables

Servings:4
Cooking Time:35 Minutes
Ingredients:
- ½ pound carrots, peeled and sliced
- 1 pound yellow squash, sliced
- 1 pound zucchini, sliced
- 1 tablespoon tarragon leaves, chopped
- 6 teaspoons olive oil, divided
- 1 teaspoon kosher salt
- ½ teaspoon ground white pepper

Directions:
1. Preheat the Air fryer to 400 °F and grease an Air fryer basket.
2. Mix 2 teaspoons olive oil and carrots in a bowl until combined.
3. Transfer into the Air fryer basket and cook for about 5 minutes.
4. Meanwhile, mix remaining 4 teaspoons of olive oil, yellow squash, zucchini, salt and white pepper in a large bowl.

5. Transfer this veggie mixture into the Air fryer basket with carrots.
6. Cook for about 30 minutes and dish out in a bowl.
7. Top with tarragon leaves and mix well to serve.

191.Baked Polenta With Chili-cheese

Servings:3
Cooking Time: 10 Minutes
Ingredients:
- 1 commercial polenta roll, sliced
- 1 cup cheddar cheese sauce
- 1 tablespoon chili powder

Directions:
1. Place the baking dish accessory in the air fryer.
2. Arrange the polenta slices in the baking dish.
3. Add the chili powder and cheddar cheese sauce.
4. Close the air fryer and cook for 10 minutes at 390°F.

192.Crispy Vegetarian Ravioli

Servings:4
Cooking Time: 6 Minutes
Ingredients:
- ¼ cup aquafaba
- ½ cup panko bread crumbs
- 1 teaspoon dried basil
- 1 teaspoon dried oregano
- 1 teaspoon garlic powder
- 2 teaspoons nutritional yeast
- 8-ounces vegan ravioli
- cooking spray
- salt and pepper to taste

Directions:
1. Line the air fryer basket with aluminum foil and brush with oil.
2. Preheat the air fryer to 400°F.
3. Mix together the panko bread crumbs, nutritional yeast, basil, oregano, and garlic powder. Season with salt and pepper to taste.
4. In another bowl, place the aquafaba.
5. Dip the ravioli in the aquafaba the dredge in the panko mixture.
6. Spray with cooking oil and place in the air fryer.
7. Cook for 6 minutes making sure that you shake the air fryer basket halfway.

193.Garlic-roasted Brussels Sprouts With Mustard

Servings: 3
Cooking Time: 20 Minutes
Ingredients:
- 1 pound Brussels sprouts, halved

- 2 tablespoons olive oil
- Sea salt and freshly ground black pepper, to taste
- 2 garlic cloves, minced
- 1 tablespoon Dijon mustard

Directions:
1. Toss the Brussels sprouts with the olive oil, salt, black pepper, and garlic.
2. Roast in the preheated Air Fryer at 380 degrees F for 15 minutes, shaking the basket occasionally.
3. Serve with Dijon mustard and enjoy!

194.Layered Tortilla Bake

Servings:6
Cooking Time: 30 Minutes
Ingredients:
- 1 (15 ounce) can black beans, rinsed and drained
- 1 cup salsa
- 1 cup salsa, divided
- 1/2 cup chopped tomatoes
- 1/2 cup sour cream
- 2 (15 ounce) cans pinto beans, drained and rinsed
- 2 cloves garlic, minced
- 2 cups shredded reduced-fat Cheddar cheese
- 2 tablespoons chopped fresh cilantro
- 7 (8 inch) flour tortillas

Directions:
1. Mash pinto beans in a large bowl and mix in garlic and salsa.
2. In another bowl whisk together tomatoes, black beans, cilantro, and ¼ cup salsa.
3. Lightly grease baking pan of air fryer with cooking spray. Spread 1 tortilla, spread ¾ cup pinto bean mixture evenly up to ½-inch away from the edge of tortilla, spread ¼ cup cheese on top. Cover with another tortilla, spread 2/3 cup black bean mixture, and then ¼ cup cheese. Repeat twice the layering process. Cover with the last tortilla, top with pinto bean mixture and then cheese.
4. Cover pan with foil.
5. Cook for 25 minutes at 390 °F, remove foil and cook for 5 minutes or until tops are lightly browned.
6. Serve and enjoy.

195.Oatmeal Stuffed Bell Pepper

Servings:2
Cooking Time:16 Minutes
Ingredients:
- 1 large red bell pepper, halved and seeded
- 1 cup cooked oatmeal
- 2 tablespoons canned red kidney beans
- 2 tablespoons plain yogurt

- 1/8 teaspoon ground cumin
- 1/8 teaspoon smoked paprika
- Salt and black pepper, to taste

Directions:
1. Preheat the Air fryer to 355 °F and grease an Air fryer pan.
2. Put the bell peppers in the Air fryer pan and cook for about 8 minutes.
3. Meanwhile, mix oatmeal with remaining ingredients in a bowl.
4. Stuff the oatmeal mixture in each pepper half and cook for about 8 minutes.
5. Dish out in a bowl and serve warm.

196.Low-calorie Beets Dish

Servings:2
Cooking Time: 20 Minutes
Ingredients:
- ⅓ cup balsamic vinegar
- 1 tbsp olive oil
- 1 tbsp honey
- Salt and pepper to taste
- 2 springs rosemary

Directions:
1. In a bowl, mix rosemary, pepper, salt, vinegar and honey. Cover beets with the prepared sauce and then coat with oil. Preheat your air fryer to 400 F, and cook the beets in the air fryer for 10 minutes. Pour the balsamic vinegar in a pan over medium heat; bring to a boil and cook until reduced by half. Drizzle the beets with balsamic glaze, to serve.

197.Rich And Easy Vegetable Croquettes

Servings: 4
Cooking Time: 15 Minutes
Ingredients:
- 1/2 pound broccoli florets
- 1 tablespoon ground flaxseeds
- 1 yellow onion, finely chopped
- 1 bell pepper, seeded and chopped
- 2 garlic cloves, pressed
- 1 teaspoon turmeric powder
- 1/2 teaspoon ground cumin
- 1/2 cup almond flour
- 1/2 cup parmesan cheese
- 2 eggs, whisked
- Salt and ground black pepper, to taste
- 2 tablespoons olive oil

Directions:
1. Blanch the broccoli in salted boiling water until al dente, about 3 to 4 minutes. Drain well and transfer to a mixing bowl; mash the broccoli florets with the remaining ingredients.
2. Form the mixture into patties and place them in the lightly greased Air Fryer basket.

3. Cook at 400 degrees F for 6 minutes, turning them over halfway through the cooking time; work in batches.
4. Serve warm with mayonnaise. Enjoy!

198.Green Beans And Mushroom Casserole

Servings:6
Cooking Time:12 Minutes
Ingredients:
- 24 ounces fresh green beans, trimmed
- 2 cups fresh button mushrooms, sliced
- 1/3 cup French fried onions
- 3 tablespoons olive oil
- 2 tablespoons fresh lemon juice
- 1 teaspoon ground sage
- 1 teaspoon garlic powder
- 1 teaspoon onion powder
- Salt and black pepper, to taste

Directions:
1. Preheat the Air fryer to 400 °F and grease an Air fryer basket.
2. Mix the green beans, mushrooms, oil, lemon juice, sage, and spices in a bowl and toss to coat well.
3. Arrange the green beans mixture into the Air fryer basket and cook for about 12 minutes.
4. Dish out in a serving dish and top with fried onions to serve.

199.Easy Baked Root Veggies

Servings:4
Cooking Time: 45 Minutes
Ingredients:
- ¼ cup olive oil
- 1 head broccoli, cut into florets
- 1 tablespoon dry onion powder
- 2 sweet potatoes, peeled and cubed
- 4 carrots, cut into chunks
- 4 zucchinis, sliced thickly
- salt and pepper to taste

Directions:
1. Preheat the air fryer to 400°F.
2. In a baking dish that can fit inside the air fryer, mix all the ingredients and bake for 45 minutes or until the vegetables are tender and the sides have browned.

200.Dilled Zucchini And Spinach Croquettes

Servings: 6
Cooking Time: 9 Minutes
Ingredients:
- 4 eggs, slightly beaten
- 1/2 cup almond flour
- 1/2 cup goat cheese, crumbled
- 1 teaspoon fine sea salt
- 4 garlic cloves, minced

- 1 cup baby spinach
- 1/2 cup parmesan cheese grated
- 1/3 teaspoon red pepper flakes
- 1 pound zucchini, peeled and grated
- 1/3 teaspoon dried dill weed

Directions:
1. Thoroughly combine all ingredients in a bowl. Now, roll the mixture to form small croquettes.
2. Air fry at 335 degrees F for 7 minutes or until golden. Tate, adjust for seasonings and serve warm.

201.Brussel Sprout Salad

Servings:4
Cooking Time:15 Minutes
Ingredients:
- 1 pound fresh medium Brussels sprouts, trimmed and halved vertically
- 2 apples, cored and chopped
- 1 red onion, sliced
- 4 cups lettuce, torn
- 3 teaspoons olive oil
- Salt and ground black pepper, as required
- For Dressing
- 2 tablespoons extra-virgin olive oil
- 2 tablespoons fresh lemon juice
- 1 tablespoon apple cider vinegar
- 1 tablespoon honey
- 1 teaspoon Dijon mustard
- Salt and ground black pepper, as required

Directions:
1. Preheat the Air fryer to 360 °F and grease an Air fryer basket.
2. Mix Brussels sprout, oil, salt, and black pepper in a bowl and toss to coat well.
3. Arrange the Brussels sprouts in the Air fryer basket and cook for about 15 minutes, flipping once in between.
4. Dish out the Brussel sprouts in a serving bowl and keep aside to cool.
5. Add apples, onion, and lettuce and mix well.
6. Mix all the ingredients for dressing in a bowl and pour over the salad.
7. Toss to coat well and serve immediately.

202.Cauliflower With Cholula Sauce

Servings: 4
Cooking Time: 20 Minutes
Ingredients:
- 1/2 cup almond flour
- 2 tablespoons flaxseed meal
- 1/2 cup water
- Salt, to taste
- 1/2 teaspoon ground black pepper
- 1/2 teaspoon shallot powder
- 1/2 teaspoon garlic powder
- 1/2 teaspoon cayenne pepper
- 2 tablespoons olive oil

- 1 pound cauliflower, broken into small florets
- 1/4 cup Cholula sauce

Directions:
1. Start by preheating your Air Fryer to 400 degrees F. Lightly grease a baking pan with cooking spray.
2. In a mixing bowl, combine the almond flour, flaxseed meal, water, spices, and olive oil. Coat the cauliflower with the prepared batter; arrange the cauliflower on the baking pan.
3. Then, bake in the preheated Air Fryer for 8 minutes or until golden brown.
4. Brush the Cholula sauce all over the cauliflower florets and bake an additional 4 to 5 minutes. Bon appétit!

203. Vegetable Casserole With Swiss Cheese

Servings: 6
Cooking Time: 40 Minutes
Ingredients:
- 1 tablespoon olive oil
- 1 shallot, sliced
- 2 cloves garlic, minced
- 1 red bell pepper, seeded and sliced
- 1 yellow bell pepper, seeded and sliced
- 1 ½ cups kale
- 1 pound broccoli florets, steamed
- 6 eggs
- 1/2 cup milk
- Sea salt and ground black pepper, to your liking
- 1 cup Swiss cheese, shredded
- 4 tablespoons Romano cheese, grated

Directions:
1. Heat the olive oil in a saucepan over medium-high heat. Sauté the shallot, garlic, and peppers for 2 to 3 minutes. Add the kale and cook until wilted.
2. Arrange the broccoli florets evenly over the bottom of a lightly greased casserole dish. Spread the sautéed mixture over the top.
3. In a mixing bowl, thoroughly combine the eggs, milk, salt, pepper, and shredded cheese. Pour the mixture into the casserole dish.
4. Lastly, top with Romano cheese. Bake at 330 degrees F for 30 minutes or until top is golden brown. Bon appétit!

204. Swiss Cheese And Eggplant Crisps

Servings: 4
Cooking Time: 45 Minutes
Ingredients:
- 1/2 pound eggplant, sliced
- 1/4 cup almond meal
- 2 tablespoons flaxseed meal

- Coarse sea salt and ground black pepper, to taste
- 1 teaspoon paprika
- 1 cup parmesan, freshly grated

Directions:
1. Toss the eggplant with 1 tablespoon of salt and let it stand for 30 minutes. Drain and rinse well.
2. Mix the almond meal, flaxseed meal, salt, black pepper, and paprika in a bowl. Then, pour in the water and whisk to combine well.
3. Then, place parmesan in another shallow bowl.
4. Dip the eggplant slices in the almond meal mixture, then in parmesan; press to coat on all sides. Transfer to the lightly greased Air Fryer basket.
5. Cook at 370 degrees F for 6 minutes. Turn each slice over and cook an additional 5 minutes.
6. Serve garnished with spicy ketchup if desired. Bon appétit!

205. Barbecue Tofu With Green Beans

Servings: 3
Cooking Time: 1 Hour
Ingredients:
- 12 ounces super firm tofu, pressed and cubed
- 1/4 cup ketchup
- 1 tablespoon white vinegar
- 1 tablespoon coconut sugar
- 1 tablespoon mustard
- 1/4 teaspoon ground black pepper
- 1/2 teaspoon sea salt
- 1/4 teaspoon smoked paprika
- 1/2 teaspoon freshly grated ginger
- 2 cloves garlic, minced
- 2 tablespoons olive oil
- 1 pound green beans

Directions:
1. Toss the tofu with the ketchup, white vinegar, coconut sugar, mustard, black pepper, sea salt, paprika, ginger, garlic, and olive oil. Let it marinate for 30 minutes.
2. Cook at 360 degrees F for 10 minutes; turn them over and cook for 12 minutes more. Reserve.
3. Place the green beans in the lightly greased Air Fryer basket. Roast at 400 degrees F for 5 minutes. Bon appétit!

206. Hummus Mushroom Pizza

Servings: 4
Cooking Time: 6 Minutes
Ingredients:
- 4 Portobello mushroom caps, stemmed and gills removed

- 1 tablespoon balsamic vinegar
- Salt and ground black pepper, as required
- 4 tablespoons pasta sauce
- 1 garlic clove, minced
- 3 ounces zucchini, shredded
- 2 tablespoons sweet red pepper, seeded and chopped
- 4 Kalamata olives, sliced
- 1 teaspoon dried basil
- ½ cup hummus

Directions:
1. Coat both sides of each mushroom cap with vinegar.
2. Now, sprinkle the inside of each mushroom cap with salt and black pepper.
3. Place one tablespoon of pasta sauce inside each mushroom and sprinkle with garlic.
4. Set the temperature of air fryer to 330 degrees F. Grease an air fryer basket.
5. Arrange mushroom caps into the prepared air fryer basket.
6. Air fry for about 3 minutes.
7. Remove from the air fryer and top each mushroom cap with zucchini, peppers and olives.
8. Then, sprinkle with basil, salt, and black pepper.
9. Place back mushroom caps into the air fryer basket.
10. Air fry for about 3 more minutes.
11. Remove from air fryer and transfer the mushrooms onto a serving platter.
12. Top each mushroom pizza with hummus and serve.

207.Croissant Rolls

Servings:8
Cooking Time: 6 Minutes
Ingredients:
- 1 (8-ounces) can croissant rolls
- 4 tablespoons butter, melted

Directions:
1. Set the temperature of air fryer to 320 degrees F. Grease an air fryer basket.
2. Arrange croissant rolls into the prepared air fryer basket.
3. Air fry for about 4 minutes.
4. Flip the side and air fry for 1-2 more minutes.
5. Remove from the air fryer and transfer onto a platter.
6. Drizzle with the melted butter and serve hot.

208.Rainbow Roasted Vegetables

Servings: 4
Cooking Time: 25 Minutes
Ingredients:

- 1 red bell pepper, seeded and cut into 1/2-inch chunks
- 1 cup squash, peeled and cut into 1/2-inch chunks
- 1 yellow bell pepper, seeded and cut into 1/2-inch chunks
- 1 yellow onion, quartered
- 1 green bell pepper, seeded and cut into 1/2-inch chunks
- 1 cup broccoli, broken into 1/2-inch florets
- 2 parsnips, trimmed and cut into 1/2-inch chunks
- 2 garlic cloves, minced
- Pink Himalayan salt and ground black pepper, to taste
- 1/2 teaspoon marjoram
- 1/2 teaspoon dried oregano
- 1/4 cup dry white wine
- 1/4 cup vegetable broth
- 1/2 cup Kalamata olives, pitted and sliced

Directions:
1. Arrange your vegetables in a single layer in the baking pan in the order of the rainbow (red, orange, yellow, and green. Scatter the minced garlic around the vegetables.
2. Season with salt, black pepper, marjoram, and oregano. Drizzle the white wine and vegetable broth over the vegetables.
3. Roast in the preheated Air Fryer at 390 degrees F for 15 minutes, rotating the pan once or twice.
4. Scatter the Kalamata olives all over your vegetables and serve warm. Bon appétit!

209.Celeriac With Greek Yogurt Dip

Servings: 2
Cooking Time: 25 Minutes
Ingredients:
- 1/2 pound celeriac, cut into 1 1/2-inch pieces
- 1 red onion, cut into 1 1/2-inch pieces
- 1 tablespoon sesame oil
- 1/2 teaspoon ground black pepper, to taste
- 1/2 teaspoon sea salt
- Spiced Yogurt:
- 1/4 cup Greek yogurt
- 2 tablespoons mayonnaise
- 1/2 teaspoon mustard seeds
- 1/2 teaspoon chili powder

Directions:
1. Place the vegetables in a single layer in the lightly greased cooking basket. Drizzle the sesame oil over vegetables.
2. Sprinkle with black pepper and sea salt.
3. Cook at 390 degrees F for 20 minutes, shaking the basket halfway through the cooking time.

4. Meanwhile, make the sauce by whisking all ingredients. Spoon the sauce over the roasted vegetables. Bon appétit!

210.Sweet 'n Nutty Marinated Cauliflower-tofu

Servings:2
Cooking Time: 20 Minutes
Ingredients:
- ¼ cup brown sugar
- ¼ cup low sodium soy sauce
- ½ teaspoon chili garlic sauce
- 1 package extra firm tofu, pressed to release extra water and cut into cubes
- 1 small head cauliflower, cut into florets
- 1 tablespoon sesame oil
- 2 ½ tablespoons almond butter
- 2 cloves of garlic, minced

Directions:
1. Place the garlic, sesame oil, soy sauce, sugar, chili garlic sauce, and almond butter in a mixing bowl. Whisk until well combined.
2. Place the tofu cubes and cauliflower in the marinade and allow to soak up the sauce for at least 30 minutes.
3. Preheat the air fryer to 400°F. Add tofu and cauliflower. Coo for 20 minutes. Shake basket halfway through cooking time.
4. Meanwhile, place the remaining marinade in a saucepan and bring to a boil over medium heat. Adjust the heat to low once boiling and stir until the sauce thickens.
5. Pour the sauce over the tofu and cauliflower.
6. Serve with rice or noodles.

211.Veggie Meatballs

Servings:3
Cooking Time: 30 Minutes
Ingredients:
- 2 tbsp soy sauce
- 1 tbsp flax meal
- 2 cups cooked chickpeas
- ½ cup sweet onion, diced
- ½ cup grated carrots
- ½ cup roasted cashews
- Juice of 1 lemon
- ½ tsp turmeric
- 1 tsp cumin
- 1 tsp garlic powder
- 1 cup rolled oats

Directions:
1. Combine oil, onions, and carrots into a baking dish and cook in the air fryer for 6 minutes at 350 F.
2. Meanwhile, ground the oats and cashews in a food processor. Place them in a large bowl. Process the chickpeas with the lemon juice and soy sauce, until smooth. Add them to the bowl as well.

3. Add onions and carrots to the chickpeas. Stir in the remaining ingredients; mix well. Make meatballs out of the mixture. Increase the temperature to 370 F and cook for 12 minutes, shaking once.

212.Herby Veggie Cornish Pasties

Servings:4
Cooking Time: 30 Minutes
Ingredients:
- ¼ cup mushrooms, chopped
- ¾ cup cold coconut oil
- 1 ½ cups plain flour
- 1 medium carrot, chopped
- 1 medium potato, diced
- 1 onion, sliced
- 1 stick celery, chopped
- 1 tablespoon nutritional yeast
- 1 tablespoon olive oil
- 1 teaspoon oregano
- a pinch of salt
- cold water for mixing the dough
- salt and pepper to taste

Directions:
1. Preheat the air fryer to 400°F.
2. Prepare the dough by mixing the flour, coconut oil, and salt in a bowl. Use a fork and press the flour to combine everything. Gradually add a drop of water to the dough until you achieve a stiff consistency of the dough. Cover the dough with a cling film and let it rest for 30 minutes inside the fridge.
3. Roll the dough out and cut into squares. Set aside.
4. Heat olive oil over medium heat and sauté the onions for 2 minutes. Add the celery, carrots and potatoes. Continue stirring for 3 to 5 minutes before adding the mushrooms and oregano.
5. Season with salt and pepper to taste. Add nutritional yeast last. Let it cool and set aside.
6. Drop a tablespoon of vegetable mixture on to the dough and seal the edges of the dough with water.
7. Place inside the air fryer basket and cook for 20 minutes or until the dough is crispy.

213.Onion Rings With Spicy Ketchup

Servings: 2
Cooking Time: 30 Minutes
Ingredients:
- 1 onion, sliced into rings
- 1/3 cup all-purpose flour
- 1/2 cup oat milk
- 1 teaspoon curry powder
- 1 teaspoon cayenne pepper
- Salt and ground black pepper, to your liking

- 1/2 cup cornmeal
- 4 tablespoons vegan parmesan
- 1/4 cup spicy ketchup

Directions:
1. Place the onion rings in the bowl with cold water; let them soak approximately 20 minutes; drain the onion rings and pat dry using a kitchen towel.
2. In a shallow bowl, mix the flour, milk, curry powder, cayenne pepper, salt, and black pepper. Mix to combine well.
3. Mix the cornmeal and vegan parmesan in another shallow bowl. Dip the onion rings in the flour/milk mixture; then, dredge in the cornmeal mixture.
4. Spritz the Air Fryer basket with cooking spray; arrange the breaded onion rings in the Air Fryer basket.
5. Cook in the preheated Air Fryer at 400 degrees F for 4 to 5 minutes, turning them over halfway through the cooking time. Serve with spicy ketchup. Bon appétit!

214.Greek-style Stuffed Peppers

Servings:4
Cooking Time: 20 Minutes
Ingredients:
- 2 cups cooked rice
- 1 onion, chopped
- 1 tbsp Greek seasoning
- ¼ cup sliced kalamata olives
- ¾ cup tomato sauce
- Salt and black pepper to taste
- 1 cup feta cheese, crumbled
- 2 tbsp fresh dill, chopped

Directions:
1. Preheat the Air fryer to 360 F. Microwave the bell peppers for 1-2 minutes until soft.
2. In a bowl, combine rice, onion, greek seasoning, feta cheese, olives, tomato sauce, salt, and pepper. Divide the mixture between the bell peppers and arrange them on a greased baking dish. Place in the air fryer and cook for 15 minutes. When ready, remove to a serving plate, scatter with dill and serve.

215.Stuffed Tomatoes

Servings:4
Cooking Time: 22 Minutes
Ingredients:
- 4 tomatoes
- 1 teaspoon olive oil
- 1 carrot, peeled and finely chopped
- 1 onion, chopped
- 1 cup frozen peas, thawed
- 1 garlic clove, minced
- 2 cups cold cooked rice
- 1 tablespoon soy sauce

Directions:
1. Cut the top of each tomato and scoop out pulp and seeds.
2. In a skillet, heat oil over low heat and sauté the carrot, onion, garlic, and peas for about 2 minutes.
3. Stir in the soy sauce and rice and remove from heat.
4. Set the temperature of air fryer to 355 degrees F. Grease an air fryer basket.
5. Stuff each tomato with the rice mixture.
6. Arrange tomatoes into the prepared air fryer basket.
7. Air fry for about 20 minutes.
8. Remove from air fryer and transfer the tomatoes onto a serving platter.
9. Set aside to cool slightly.
10. Serve warm.

216.Crispy Vegie Tempura Style

Servings:3
Cooking Time:15 Minutes
Ingredients:
- ¼ teaspoon salt
- ¾ cup club soda
- 1 ½ cups panko break crumbs
- 1 cup broccoli florets
- 1 egg, beaten
- 1 red bell pepper, cut into strips
- 1 small sweet potato, peeled and cut into thick slices
- 1 small zucchini, cut into thick slices
- 1/3 cup all-purpose flour
- 2/3 cup cornstarch
- Non-stick cooking spray

Directions:
1. Dredge the vegetables in a cornstarch and all-purpose flour mixture.
2. Once all vegetables are dusted with flour, dip each vegetable in a mixture of egg and club soda before dredging in bread crumbs.
3. Place the vegetables on the double layer rack accessory and spray with cooking oil.
4. Place inside the air fryer.
5. Close and cook for 20 minutes at 330°F.

217.Fried Falafel Recipe From The Middle East

Servings:8
Cooking Time: 15 Minutes
Ingredients:
- ¼ cup coriander, chopped
- ¼ cup parsley, chopped
- ½ onion, diced
- ½ teaspoon coriander seeds
- ½ teaspoon red pepper flakes
- ½ teaspoon salt
- 1 tablespoon juice from freshly squeezed lemon

- 1 teaspoon cumin seeds
- 2 cups chickpeas from can, drained and rinsed
- 3 cloves garlic
- 3 tablespoons all-purpose flour
- cooking spray

Directions:
1. In a skillet over medium heat, toast the cumin and coriander seeds until fragrant.
2. Place the toasted seeds in a mortar and grind the seeds.
3. In a food processor, place all ingredients except for the cooking spray. Add the toasted cumin and coriander seeds.
4. Pulse until fine.
5. Shape the mixture into falafels and spray cooking oil.
6. Place inside a preheated air fryer and make sure that they do not overlap.
7. Cook at 400°F for 15 minutes or until the surface becomes golden brown.

218.Baked Portobello, Pasta 'n Cheese

Servings:4
Cooking Time: 30 Minutes
Ingredients:
- 1 cup milk
- 1 cup shredded mozzarella cheese
- 1 large clove garlic, minced
- 1 tablespoon vegetable oil
- 1/4 cup margarine
- 1/4 teaspoon dried basil
- 1/4-pound portobello mushrooms, thinly sliced
- 2 tablespoons all-purpose flour
- 2 tablespoons soy sauce
- 4-ounce penne pasta, cooked according to manufacturer's Directions for Cooking
- 5-ounce frozen chopped spinach, thawed

Directions:
1. Lightly grease baking pan of air fryer with oil. For 2 minutes, heat on 360 °F. Add mushrooms and cook for a minute. Transfer to a plate.
2. In same pan, melt margarine for a minute. Stir in basil, garlic, and flour. Cook for 3 minutes. Stir and cook for another 2 minutes. Stir in half of milk slowly while whisking continuously. Cook for another 2 minutes. Mix well. Cook for another 2 minutes. Stir in remaining milk and cook for another 3 minutes.
3. Add cheese and mix well.
4. Stir in soy sauce, spinach, mushrooms, and pasta. Mix well. Top with remaining cheese.
5. Cook for 15 minutes at 390 °F until tops are lightly browned.
6. Serve and enjoy.

219.Classic Vegan Chili

Servings: 3
Cooking Time: 40 Minutes
Ingredients:
- 1 tablespoon olive oil
- 1/2 yellow onion, chopped
- 2 garlic cloves, minced
- 2 red bell peppers, seeded and chopped
- 1 red chili pepper, seeded and minced
- Sea salt and ground black pepper, to taste
- 1 teaspoon ground cumin
- 1 teaspoon cayenne pepper
- 1 teaspoon Mexican oregano
- 1/2 teaspoon mustard seeds
- 1/2 teaspoon celery seeds
- 1 can (28-ounces) diced tomatoes with juice
- 1 cup vegetable broth
- 1 (15-ounce) can black beans, rinsed and drained
- 1 bay leaf
- 1 teaspoon cider vinegar
- 1 avocado, sliced

Directions:
1. Start by preheating your Air Fryer to 365 degrees F.
2. Heat the olive oil in a baking pan until sizzling. Then, sauté the onion, garlic, and peppers in the baking pan. Cook for 4 to 6 minutes.
3. Now, add the salt, black pepper, cumin, cayenne pepper, oregano, mustard seeds, celery seeds, tomatoes, and broth. Cook for 20 minutes, stirring every 4 minutes.
4. Stir in the canned beans, bay leaf, cider vinegar; let it cook for a further 8 minutes, stirring halfway through the cooking time.
5. Serve in individual bowls garnished with the avocado slices. Enjoy!

220.Cauliflower Rice With Tofu

Servings:4
Cooking Time: 30 Minutes
Ingredients:
- ½ block tofu
- ½ cup diced onion
- 2 tbsp soy sauce
- 1 tsp turmeric
- 1 cup diced carrot
- Cauliflower:
- 3 cups cauliflower rice (pulsed in a food processor)
- 2 tbsp soy sauce
- ½ cup chopped broccoli
- 2 garlic cloves, minced
- 1 ½ tsp toasted sesame oil
- 1 tbsp minced ginger
- ½ cup frozen peas
- 1 tbsp rice vinegar

Directions:

1. Preheat the air fryer to 370 F, crumble the tofu and combine it with all tofu ingredients. Place in a baking dish and air fry for 10 minutes. Place all cauliflower ingredients in a large bowl; mix to combine.
2. Add the cauliflower mixture to the tofu and stir to combine; cook for 12 minutes. Serve and enjoy.

221.Brown Rice, Spinach 'n Tofu Frittata

Servings:4
Cooking Time: 55 Minutes
Ingredients:

- ½ cup baby spinach, chopped
- ½ cup kale, chopped
- ½ onion, chopped
- ½ teaspoon turmeric
- 1 ¾ cups brown rice, cooked
- 1 flax egg (1 tablespoon flaxseed meal + 3 tablespoon cold water)
- 1 package firm tofu
- 1 tablespoon olive oil
- 1 yellow pepper, chopped
- 2 tablespoons soy sauce
- 2 teaspoons arrowroot powder
- 2 teaspoons Dijon mustard
- 2/3 cup almond milk
- 3 big mushrooms, chopped
- 3 tablespoons nutritional yeast
- 4 cloves garlic, crushed
- 4 spring onions, chopped
- a handful of basil leaves, chopped

Directions:

1. Preheat the air fryer to 375°F. Grease a pan that will fit inside the air fryer.
2. Prepare the frittata crust by mixing the brown rice and flax egg. Press the rice onto the baking dish until you form a crust. Brush with a little oil and cook for 10 minutes.
3. Meanwhile, heat olive oil in a skillet over medium flame and sauté the garlic and onions for 2 minutes.
4. Add the pepper and mushroom and continue stirring for 3 minutes.
5. Stir in the kale, spinach, spring onions, and basil. Remove from the pan and set aside.
6. In a food processor, pulse together the tofu, mustard, turmeric, soy sauce, nutritional yeast, vegan milk and arrowroot powder. Pour in a mixing bowl and stir in the sautéed vegetables.
7. Pour the vegan frittata mixture over the rice crust and cook in the air fryer for 40 minutes.

222.Spiced Butternut Squash

Servings:4

Cooking Time:20 Minutes
Ingredients:

- 1 medium butternut squash, peeled, seeded and cut into chunk
- 2 teaspoons cumin seeds
- 2 tablespoons pine nuts
- 2 tablespoons fresh cilantro, chopped
- 1/8 teaspoon garlic powder
- 1/8 teaspoon chili flakes, crushed
- Salt and ground black pepper, as required
- 1 tablespoon olive oil

Directions:

1. Preheat the Air fryer to 375 °F and grease an Air fryer basket.
2. Mix the squash, spices and olive oil in a bowl.
3. Arrange the butternut squash chunks into the Air fryer basket and cook for about 20 minutes.
4. Dish out the butternut squash chunks onto serving plates and serve garnished with pine nuts and cilantro.

223.Sautéed Spinach

Servings:2
Cooking Time:9 Minutes
Ingredients:

- 1 small onion, chopped
- 6 ounces fresh spinach
- 2 tablespoons olive oil
- 1 teaspoon ginger, minced
- Salt and black pepper, to taste

Directions:

1. Preheat the Air fryer to 360 °F and grease an Air fryer pan.
2. Put olive oil, onions and ginger in the Air fryer pan and place in the Air fryer basket.
3. Cook for about 4 minutes and add spinach, salt, and black pepper.
4. Cook for about 4 more minutes and dish out in a bowl to serve.

224.Open-faced Vegan Flatbread-wich

Servings:4
Cooking Time: 25 Minutes
Ingredients:

- 1 can chickpeas, drained and rinsed
- 1 medium-sized head of cauliflower, cut into florets
- 1 tablespoon extra-virgin olive oil
- 2 ripe avocados, mashed
- 2 tablespoons lemon juice
- 4 flatbreads, toasted
- salt and pepper to taste

Directions:

1. Preheat the air fryer to 425°F.
2. In a mixing bowl, combine the cauliflower, chickpeas, olive oil, and lemon juice. Season with salt and pepper to taste.

3. Place inside the air fryer basket and cook for 25 minutes.
4. Once cooked, place on half of the flatbread and add avocado mash.
5. Season with more salt and pepper to taste.
6. Serve with hot sauce.

225.Cheesy Spinach

Servings:3
Cooking Time: 15 Minutes
Ingredients:
- 1 (10-ounces) package frozen spinach, thawed
- ½ cup onion, chopped
- 2 teaspoons garlic, minced
- 4 ounces cream cheese, chopped
- ½ teaspoon ground nutmeg
- Salt and ground black pepper, as required
- ¼ cup Parmesan cheese, shredded

Directions:
1. In a bowl, mix well spinach, onion, garlic, cream cheese, nutmeg, salt, and black pepper.
2. Set the temperature of air fryer to 350 degrees F. Grease an air fryer pan.
3. Place spinach mixture into the prepared air fryer pan.
4. Air fry for about 10 minutes.
5. Remove from air fryer and stir the mixture well.
6. Sprinkle the spinach mixture evenly with Parmesan cheese.
7. Now, set the temperature of air fryer to 400 degrees F and air fry for 5 more minutes.
8. Remove from air fryer and transfer the spinach mixture onto serving plates.
9. Serve hot.

226.Rich Asparagus And Mushroom Patties

Servings: 4
Cooking Time: 15 Minutes
Ingredients:
- 3/4 pound asparagus spears
- 1 tablespoon canola oil
- 1 teaspoon paprika
- Sea salt and freshly ground black pepper, to taste
- 1 teaspoon garlic powder
- 3 tablespoons scallions, chopped
- 1 cup button mushrooms, chopped
- 1/2 cup parmesan cheese, grated
- 2 tablespoons flax seeds
- 2 eggs, beaten
- 4 tablespoons sour cream, for garnish

Directions:
1. Place the asparagus spears in the lightly greased cooking basket. Toss the asparagus

with the canola oil, paprika, salt, and black pepper.
2. Cook in the preheated Air Fryer at 400 degrees F for 5 minutes. Chop the asparagus spears and add the garlic powder, scallions, mushrooms, parmesan, flax seeds, and eggs.
3. Mix until everything is well incorporated and form the asparagus mixture into patties.
4. Cook in the preheated Air Fryer at 400 degrees F for 5 minutes, flipping halfway through the cooking time. Serve with well-chilled sour cream. Bon appétit!

227.Feisty Baby Carrots

Servings:4
Cooking Time: 20 Minutes
Ingredients:
- 1 tsp dried dill
- 1 tbsp olive oil
- 1 tbsp honey
- Salt and pepper to taste

Directions:
1. Preheat air fryer to 350 F. In a bowl, mix oil, carrots and honey; stir to coat. Season with dill, pepper and salt. Place the prepared carrots in your air fryer's cooking basket and cook for 12 minutes.

228.Ultimate Vegan Calzone

Servings: 1
Cooking Time: 25 Minutes
Ingredients:
- 1 teaspoon olive oil
- 1/2 small onion, chopped
- 2 sweet peppers, seeded and sliced
- Sea salt, to taste
- 1/4 teaspoon ground black pepper
- 1/4 teaspoon dried oregano
- 4 ounces prepared Italian pizza dough
- 1/4 cup marinara sauce
- 2 ounces plant-based cheese Mozzarella-style, shredded

Directions:
1. Heat the olive oil in a nonstick skillet. Once hot, cook the onion and peppers until tender and fragrant, about 5 minutes. Add salt, black pepper, and oregano.
2. Sprinkle some flour on a kitchen counter and roll out the pizza dough.
3. Spoon the marinara sauce over half of the dough; add the sautéed mixture and sprinkle with the vegan cheese. Now, gently fold over the dough to create a pocket; make sure to seal the edges.
4. Use a fork to poke the dough in a few spots. Add a few drizzles of olive oil and place in the lightly greased cooking basket.
5. Bake in the preheated Air Fryer at 330 degrees F for 12 minutes, turning the

calzones over halfway through the cooking time. Bon appétit!

229. Eggplant Steaks With Garlic & Parsley

Servings:4
Cooking Time: 20 Minutes
Ingredients:
- 2 cups breadcrumbs
- 1 tsp Italian seasoning
- 1 cup flour
- Salt to taste
- 4 eggs
- 2 garlic cloves, sliced
- 2 tbsp parsley, chopped

Directions:
1. Preheat the Air fryer to 390 F. Grease the air fryer basket with cooking spray.
2. In a bowl, beat the eggs with salt. In a separate bowl, mix breadcrumbs and Italian seasoning. In a third bowl, pour the flour. Dip eggplant steaks in the flour, followed by a dip in the eggs, and finally, coat with breadcrumbs. Place the prepared steaks in your air fryer's cooking basket and cook for 10 minutes, flipping once. Remove to a platter and sprinkle with garlic and parsley to serve.

230. Shepherd's Pie Vegetarian Approved

Servings:3
Cooking Time: 35 Minutes
Directions:
1. Boil potatoes until tender. Drain and transfer to a bowl. Mash potatoes with salt, vegan cream cheese, olive oil, soy milk, and vegan mayonnaise. Mix well until smooth. Set aside.
2. Lightly grease baking pan of air fryer with cooking spray. Add carrot, celery, onions, tomato, and peas. For 10 minutes, cook on 360 °F. Stirring halfway through cooking time.
3. Stir in pepper, garlic, and Italian seasoning.
4. Stir in vegetarian ground beef substitute. Cook for 5 minutes while halfway through cooking time crumbling and mixing the beef substitute.
5. Evenly spread the beef and veggie mixture in pan. Top evenly with mashed potato mixture.
6. Cook for another 20 minutes or until mashed potatoes are lightly browned.
7. Serve and enjoy.

231. Easy Crispy Shawarma Chickpeas

Servings: 4
Cooking Time: 25 Minutes
Ingredients:
- 1 (12-ounce) can chickpeas, drained and rinsed

- 2 tablespoons canola oil
- 1 teaspoon cayenne pepper
- 1 teaspoon sea salt
- 1 tablespoon Shawarma spice blend

Directions:
1. Toss all ingredients in a mixing bowl.
2. Roast in the preheated Air Fryer at 380 degrees F for 10 minutes, shaking the basket halfway through the cooking time.
3. Work in batches. Bon appétit!

232. Extreme Zucchini Fries

Servings:4
Cooking Time: 25 Minutes
Ingredients:
- 2 egg whites
- ½ cup seasoned breadcrumbs
- 2 tbsp grated Parmesan cheese
- Cooking spray as needed
- ¼ tsp garlic powder
- Salt and pepper to taste

Directions:
1. Preheat your air fryer to 420 F, and coat cooling rack with cooking spray; place it in the fryer's basket. In a bowl, beat the egg whites and season with salt and pepper. In another bowl, mix garlic powder, cheese and breadcrumbs.
2. Take zucchini slices and dredge them in eggs, followed by breadcrumbs. Add zucchini to the rack (in the cooking basket) and spray more oil. cook for 20 minutes. Serve and enjoy!

233. Classic Onion Rings

Servings: 8
Cooking Time: 30 Minutes
Ingredients:
- 2 medium-sized yellow onions, cut into rings
- 1 cup almond flour
- 1/2 teaspoon baking soda
- 1 teaspoon baking powder
- 1 ½ teaspoons sea salt flakes
- 2 medium-sized eggs
- 1 ½ cups plain milk
- 1 ¼ cups grated parmesan cheese
- 1/2 teaspoon green peppercorns, freshly cracked
- 1/2 teaspoon dried dill weed
- 1/4 teaspoon paprika

Directions:
1. Begin by preheating your Air Fryer to 356 degrees F.
2. Place the onion rings into the bowl with icy cold water; let them stay 15 to 20 minutes; drain the onion rings and dry them using a kitchen towel.

3. In a shallow bowl, mix the flour together with baking soda, baking powder and sea salt flakes. Then, coat each onion ring with the flour mixture;
4. In another shallow bowl, beat the eggs with milk; add the mixture to the remaining flour mixture and whisk well. Dredge the coated onion rings into this batter.
5. In a third bowl, mix the parmesan cheese, green peppercorns, dill, and paprika. Roll the onion rings over the parmesan cheese mixture, covering well.
6. Air-fry them in the cooking basket for 8 to 11 minutes or until thoroughly cooked to golden.

234.Zucchini With Mediterranean Dill Sauce

Servings: 4
Cooking Time: 1 Hour
Ingredients:
- 1 pound zucchini, peeled and cubed
- 2 tablespoons melted butter
- 1 teaspoon sea salt flakes
- 1 sprig rosemary, leaves only, crushed
- 2 sprigs thyme, leaves only, crushed
- 1/2 teaspoon freshly cracked black peppercorns
- For Mediterranean Dipping Sauce:
- 1/2 cup mascarpone cheese
- 1/3 cup yogurt
- 1 tablespoon fresh dill, chopped
- 1 tablespoon olive oil

Directions:
1. Firstly, set your Air Fryer to cook at 350 degrees F. Now, add the potato cubes to the bowl with cold water and soak them approximately for 35 minutes.
2. After that, dry the potato cubes using a paper towel.
3. In a mixing dish, thoroughly whisk the melted butter with sea salt flakes, rosemary, thyme, and freshly cracked peppercorns. Rub the potato cubes with this butter/spice mix.
4. Air-fry the potato cubes in the cooking basket for 18 to 20 minutes or until cooked through; make sure to shake the potatoes to cook them evenly.
5. Meanwhile, make the Mediterranean dipping sauce by mixing the remaining ingredients. Serve warm potatoes with Mediterranean sauce for dipping and enjoy!

235.Thai Sweet Potato Balls

Servings: 4
Cooking Time: 50 Minutes
Ingredients:
- 1 pound sweet potatoes

- 1 cup brown sugar
- 1 tablespoon orange juice
- 2 teaspoons orange zest
- 1/2 teaspoon ground cinnamon
- 1/4 teaspoon ground cloves
- 1/2 cup almond meal
- 1 teaspoon baking powder
- 1 cup coconut flakes

Directions:
1. Bake the sweet potatoes at 380 degrees F for 30 to 35 minutes until tender; peel and mash them.
2. Add the brown sugar, orange juice, orange zest, ground cinnamon, cloves, almond meal, and baking powder; mix to combine well.
3. Roll the balls in the coconut flakes.
4. Bake in the preheated Air Fryer at 360 degrees F for 15 minutes or until thoroughly cooked and crispy.
5. Repeat the process until you run out of ingredients. Bon appétit!

236.Drizzling Blooming Onion

Servings:4
Cooking Time: 20 Minutes
Ingredients:
- Olive oil as needed
- 1 tsp cayenne pepper
- 1 tsp garlic powder
- 2 cups flour
- 1 tbsp pepper
- 1 tbsp paprika
- 1 tbsp salt
- ¼ cup mayonnaise
- 1 tbsp ketchup
- ¼ cup mayonnaise
- ¼ cup sour cream

Directions:
1. In a bowl, mix salt, pepper, paprika, flour, garlic powder, and cayenne pepper. Add mayonnaise, ketchup, sour cream to the mixture and stir. Coat the onions with prepared mixture and spray with oil. Preheat your air fryer to 360 F. Add the coated onions to the basket and cook for 15 minutes.

237.Crispy Ham Rolls

Servings:3
Cooking Time: 17 Minutes
Ingredients:
- 3 packages Pepperidge farm rolls
- 1 tbsp softened butter
- 1 tsp mustard seeds
- 1 tsp poppy seeds
- 1 small chopped onion

Directions:
1. Mix butter, mustard, onion and poppy seeds. Spread the mixture on top of the rolls. Cover

with the chopped ham. Roll up and arrange them on the basket of the air fryer; cook at 350 F for 15 minutes.

238.Eggplant Caviar

Servings:3
Cooking Time: 20 Minutes
Ingredients:

- ½ red onion, chopped and blended
- 2 tbsp balsamic vinegar
- 1 tbsp olive oil
- salt

Directions:

1. Arrange the eggplants in the basket and cook them for 15 minutes at 380 F. Remove them and let them cool. Then cut the eggplants in half, lengthwise, and empty their insides with a spoon.
2. Blend the onion in a blender. Put the inside of the eggplants in the blender and process everything. Add the vinegar, olive oil and salt, then blend again. Serve cool with bread and tomato sauce or ketchup.

239.Crispy Leek Strips

Servings: 6
Cooking Time: 52 Minutes
Ingredients:

- 1/2 teaspoon porcini powder
- 1 cup almond flour
- 1/2 cup coconut flour
- 1 tablespoon vegetable oil
- 2 medium-sized leeks, slice into julienne strips
- 2 large-sized dishes with ice water
- 2 teaspoons onion powder
- Fine sea salt and cayenne pepper, to taste

Directions:

1. Allow the leeks to soak in ice water for about 25 minutes; drain well.
2. Place the flour, salt, cayenne pepper, onions powder, and porcini powder into a resealable bag. Add the leeks and shake to coat well.
3. Drizzle vegetable oil over the seasoned leeks. Air fry at 390 degrees F for about 18 minutes; turn them halfway through the cooking time.
4. Serve with homemade mayonnaise or any other sauce for dipping. Enjoy!

240.Paprika Brussels Sprout Chips

Servings: 2
Cooking Time: 20 Minutes
Ingredients:

- 10 Brussels sprouts
- 1 teaspoon canola oil
- 1 teaspoon coarse sea salt
- 1 teaspoon paprika

Directions:

1. Toss all ingredients in the lightly greased Air Fryer basket.
2. Bake at 380 degrees F for 15 minutes, shaking the basket halfway through the cooking time to ensure even cooking.
3. Serve and enjoy!

241.Garden Fresh Green Beans

Servings:4
Cooking Time:12 Minutes
Ingredients:

- 1 pound green beans, washed and trimmed
- 1 teaspoon butter, melted
- 1 tablespoon fresh lemon juice
- ¼ teaspoon garlic powder
- Salt and freshly ground pepper, to taste

Directions:

1. Preheat the Air fryer to 400 °F and grease an Air fryer basket.
2. Put all the ingredients in a large bowl and transfer into the Air fryer basket.
3. Cook for about 8 minutes and dish out in a bowl to serve warm.

242.Curly Vegan Fries

Servings:2
Cooking Time: 20 Minutes
Ingredients:

- 1 tbsp tomato ketchup
- 2 tbsp olive oil
- Salt and pepper to taste
- 2 tbsp coconut oil

Directions:

1. Preheat your air fryer to 360 F and use a spiralizer to spiralize the potatoes. In a bowl, mix oil, coconut oil, salt and pepper. Cover the potatoes with the oil mixture. Place the potatoes in the cooking basket and cook for 15 minutes. Serve with ketchup and enjoy!

243.Pesto Tomatoes

Servings:4
Cooking Time: 16 Minutes
Ingredients:

- For Pesto:
- ½ cup plus 1 tablespoon olive oil, divided
- 3 tablespoons pine nuts
- Salt, to taste
- ½ cup fresh basil, chopped
- ½ cup fresh parsley, chopped
- 1 garlic clove, chopped
- ½ cup Parmesan cheese, grated
- For Tomatoes:
- 2 heirloom tomatoes, cut into ½ inch thick slices
- 8 ounces feta cheese, cut into ½ inch thick slices.

- ½ cup red onions, thinly sliced
- 1 tablespoon olive oil
- Salt, to taste

Directions:
1. Set the temperature of air fryer to 390 degrees F. Grease an air fryer basket.
2. In a bowl, mix together one tablespoon of oil, pine nuts and pinch of salt.
3. Arrange pine nuts into the prepared air fryer basket.
4. Air fry for about 1-2 minutes.
5. Remove from air fryer and transfer the pine nuts onto a paper towel-lined plate.
6. In a food processor, add the toasted pine nuts, fresh herbs, garlic, Parmesan, and salt and pulse until just combined.
7. While motor is running, slowly add the remaining oil and pulse until smooth.
8. Transfer into a bowl, covered and refrigerate until serving.
9. Spread about one tablespoon of pesto onto each tomato slice.
10. Top each tomato slice with one feta and onion slice and drizzle with oil.
11. Arrange tomato slices into the prepared air fryer basket in a single layer.
12. Air fry for about 12-14 minutes.
13. Remove from air fryer and transfer the tomato slices onto serving plates.
14. Sprinkle with a little salt and serve with the remaining pesto.

244.Stuffed Okra

Servings:2
Cooking Time:12 Minutes
Ingredients:
- 8 ounces large okra
- ¼ cup chickpea flour
- ¼ of onion, chopped
- 2 tablespoons coconut, grated freshly
- 1 teaspoon garam masala powder
- ½ teaspoon ground turmeric
- ½ teaspoon red chili powder
- ½ teaspoon ground cumin
- Salt, to taste

Directions:
1. Preheat the Air fryer to 390 °F and grease an Air fryer basket.
2. Mix the flour, onion, grated coconut, and spices in a bowl and toss to coat well.
3. Stuff the flour mixture into okra and arrange into the Air fryer basket.
4. Cook for about 12 minutes and dish out in a serving plate.

POULTRY RECIPES

245. Parsley Duck

Servings: 4
Cooking Time: 25 Minutes
Ingredients:
- 4 duck breast fillets, boneless, skin-on and scored
- 2 tablespoons olive oil
- 2 tablespoons parsley, chopped
- Salt and black pepper to the taste
- 1 cup chicken stock
- 1 teaspoon balsamic vinegar

Directions:
1. Heat up a pan that fits your air fryer with the oil over medium heat, add the duck breasts skin side down and sear for 5 minutes. Add the rest of the ingredients, toss, put the pan in the fryer and cook at 380 degrees F for 20 minutes. Divide everything between plates and serve

246. Chicken With Mushrooms

Servings: 4
Cooking Time: 24 Minutes
Ingredients:
- 2 lbs chicken breasts, halved
- 1/3 cup sun-dried tomatoes
- 8 oz mushrooms, sliced
- 1/2 cup mayonnaise
- 1 tsp salt

Directions:
1. Preheat the air fryer to 370 F.
2. Spray air fryer baking dish with cooking spray.
3. Place chicken breasts into the baking dish and top with sun-dried tomatoes, mushrooms, mayonnaise, and salt. Mix well.
4. Place dish in the air fryer and cook for 24 minutes.
5. Serve and enjoy.

247. Tangy And Buttery Chicken

Servings: 4
Cooking Time: 20 Minutes
Ingredients:
- ½ tablespoon Worcestershire sauce
- 1 teaspoon finely grated orange zest
- 2 tablespoons melted butter
- ½ teaspoon smoked paprika
- 4 chicken drumsticks, rinsed and halved
- 1 teaspoon sea salt flakes
- 1 tablespoon cider vinegar
- 1/2 teaspoon mixed peppercorns, freshly cracked

Directions:
1. Firstly, pat the chicken drumsticks dry. Coat them with the melted butter on all sides.

Toss the chicken drumsticks with the other ingredients.
2. Transfer them to the Air Fryer cooking basket and roast for about 13 minutes at 345 degrees F. Bon appétit!

248. Chicken-parm, Broccoli 'n Mushroom Bake

Servings: 2
Cooking Time: 40 Minutes
Ingredients:
- 1 (13.5 ounce) can spinach, drained
- 1 cup shredded mozzarella cheese
- 1/2 (10.75 ounce) can condensed cream of mushroom soup
- 1/3 cup bacon bits
- 1/4 cup grated Parmesan cheese
- 1/4 cup half-and-half
- 1-1/2 teaspoons Italian seasoning
- 1-1/2 teaspoons lemon juice
- 1-1/2 teaspoons minced garlic
- 2 ounces fresh mushrooms, sliced
- 2 skinless, boneless chicken breast halves
- 2 tablespoons butter

Directions:
1. Lightly grease baking pan of air fryer with cooking spray. Add chicken breast and for 20 minutes, cook on 360 °F. Halfway through cooking time, turnover chicken breast. Once done, transfer to a plate and set aside.
2. In same baking pan, melt butter. Stir in Parmesan cheese, half and half, Italian seasoning, mushroom soup, lemon juice, and garlic. Mix well and cook for 5 minutes or until heated through.
3. Stir in spinach and chicken. Tope with bacon bits and mozzarella cheese.
4. Cook for 15 minutes at 390 °F until tops are lightly browned.
5. Serve and enjoy.

249. Spice-rubbed Jerk Chicken Wings

Servings: 4
Cooking Time: 40 Minutes
Ingredients:
- 1 tbsp olive oil
- 3 cloves garlic, minced
- 1 tbsp chili powder
- ½ tbsp cinnamon powder
- ½ tsp allspice
- 1 habanero pepper, seeded
- 1 tbsp soy sauce
- ½ tbsp white pepper
- ¼ cup red wine vinegar
- 3 tbsp lime juice
- 2 Scallions, chopped

- ½ tbsp grated ginger
- ½ tbsp chopped fresh thyme
- ⅓ tbsp sugar
- ½ tbsp salt

Directions:
1. In a bowl, add the olive oil, soy sauce, garlic, habanero pepper, allspice, cinnamon powder, cayenne pepper, white pepper, salt, sugar, thyme, ginger, scallions, lime juice, and red wine vinegar; mix well.
2. Add the chicken wings to the marinade mixture and coat it well with the mixture. Cover the bowl with cling film and refrigerate the chicken to marinate for 16 hours. Preheat the air fryer to 400 F. Remove the chicken from the fridge, drain all the liquid, and pat each wing dry using a paper towel.
3. Place half of the wings in the basket and cook for 16 minutes. Shake halfway through. Remove onto a serving platter. Serve with blue cheese dip or ranch dressing.

250.Chicken Wings

Servings: 4
Cooking Time: 55 Minutes
Ingredients:
- 3 lb. bone-in chicken wings
- ¾ cup flour
- 1 tbsp. old bay seasoning
- 4 tbsp. butter
- Couple fresh lemons

Directions:
1. In a bowl, combine the all-purpose flour and Old Bay seasoning.
2. Toss the chicken wings with the mixture to coat each one well.
3. Pre-heat the Air Fryer to 375°F.
4. Give the wings a shake to shed any excess flour and place each one in the Air Fryer. You may have to do this in multiple batches, so as to not overlap any.
5. Cook for 30 – 40 minutes, shaking the basket frequently, until the wings are cooked through and crispy.
6. In the meantime, melt the butter in a frying pan over a low heat. Squeeze one or two lemons and add the juice to the pan. Mix well.
7. Serve the wings topped with the sauce.

251.One-tray Parmesan Wings

Servings:4
Cooking Time: 30 Minutes
Ingredients:
- 1 tsp Dijon mustard
- Salt to taste
- 2 tbsp olive oil
- 2 cloves garlic, crushed

- 4 tbsp grated Parmesan cheese
- 2 tsp chopped fresh parsley

Directions:
1. Preheat the Air fryer to 380 F. Grease the air fryer basket with cooking spray.
2. Season chicken with salt and pepper. Brush it with mustard. On a plate, pour 2 tbsp of the Parmesan cheese. Coat chicken with Parmesan cheese. Drizzle with olive oil and place in the air fryer basket. Cook for 20 minutes. Top with the remaining Parmesan cheese and parsley to serve.

252.Hot Chicken Skin

Servings: 4
Cooking Time: 30 Minutes
Ingredients:
- ½ teaspoon chili paste
- 8 oz chicken skin
- 1 teaspoon sesame oil
- ½ teaspoon chili powder
- ½ teaspoon salt

Directions:
1. In the shallow bowl mix up chili paste, sesame oil, chili powder, and salt. Then brush the chicken skin with chili mixture well and leave for 10 minutes to marinate. Meanwhile, preheat the air fryer to 365F. Put the marinated chicken skin in the air fryer and cook it for 20 minutes. When the time is finished, flip the chicken skin on another side and cook it for 10 minutes more or until the chicken skin is crunchy.

253.Mediterranean Chicken Breasts With Roasted Tomatoes

Servings: 8
Cooking Time: 1 Hour
Ingredients:
- 2 teaspoons olive oil, melted
- 3 pounds chicken breasts, bone-in
- 1/2 teaspoon black pepper, freshly ground
- 1/2 teaspoon salt
- 1 teaspoon cayenne pepper
- 2 tablespoons fresh parsley, minced
- 1 teaspoon fresh basil, minced
- 1 teaspoon fresh rosemary, minced
- 4 medium-sized Roma tomatoes, halved

Directions:
1. Start by preheating your Air Fryer to 370 degrees F. Brush the cooking basket with 1 teaspoon of olive oil.
2. Sprinkle the chicken breasts with all seasonings listed above.
3. Cook for 25 minutes or until chicken breasts are slightly browned. Work in batches.

4. Arrange the tomatoes in the cooking basket and brush them with the remaining teaspoon of olive oil. Season with sea salt.
5. Cook the tomatoes at 350 degrees F for 10 minutes, shaking halfway through the cooking time. Serve with chicken breasts. Bon appétit!

254.Deliciously Crisp Chicken

Servings:4
Cooking Time:12 Minutes
Ingredients:
- 1 egg, beaten
- ½ cup breadcrumbs
- 8 skinless, boneless chicken tenderloins
- 2 tablespoons vegetable oil

Directions:
1. Preheat the Air fryer to 355 °F and grease an Air fryer basket.
2. Whisk the egg in a shallow dish and mix vegetable oil and breadcrumbs in another shallow dish.
3. Dip the chicken tenderloins in egg and then coat in the breadcrumb mixture.
4. Arrange the chicken tenderloins in the Air fryer basket and cook for about 12 minutes.
5. Dish out and serve warm.

255.Garlic Chicken Sausages

Servings: 4
Cooking Time: 10 Minutes
Ingredients:
- 1 garlic clove, diced
- 1 spring onion, chopped
- 1 cup ground chicken
- ½ teaspoon salt
- ½ teaspoon ground black pepper
- 4 sausage links
- 1 teaspoon olive oil

Directions:
1. In the mixing bowl, mix up a diced garlic clove, onion, ground chicken, salt, and ground black pepper. Then fill the sausage links with the ground chicken mixture. Cut every sausage into halves and secure the endings. Preheat the air fryer to 365. Brush the sausages with olive oil and put it in the air fryer. Cook them for 10 minutes. Then flip the sausages on another side and cook for 5 minutes more. Increase the cooking time to 390F and cook for 8 minutes for faster results.

256.Chicken Tenders

Servings: 4
Cooking Time: 30 Minutes
Ingredients:
- 1 lb. chicken tenders
- 1 tsp. ginger, minced

- 4 garlic cloves, minced
- 2 tbsp. sesame oil
- 6 tbsp. pineapple juice
- 2 tbsp. soy sauce
- ½ tsp. pepper

Directions:
1. Put all of the ingredients, except for the chicken, in a bowl and combine well.
2. Thread the chicken onto skewers and coat with the seasonings. Allow to marinate for 2 hours.
3. Pre-heat the Air Fryer to 350°F.
4. Put the marinated chicken in fryer basket and cook for 18 minutes. Serve hot.

257.Asian Spicy Turkey

Servings: 6
Cooking Time: 35 Minutes
Ingredients:
- 1 tablespoon sesame oil
- 2 pounds turkey thighs
- 1 teaspoon Chinese Five-spice powder
- 1 teaspoon pink Himalayan salt
- 1/4 teaspoon Sichuan pepper
- 1 tablespoon Chinese rice vinegar
- 2 tablespoons soy sauce
- 1 tablespoon chili sauce
- 1 tablespoon mustard

Directions:
1. Preheat your Air Fryer to 360 degrees F.
2. Brush the sesame oil all over the turkey thighs. Season them with spices.
3. Cook for 23 minutes, turning over once or twice. Make sure to work in batches to ensure even cooking
4. In the meantime, combine the remaining ingredients in a wok (or similar type pan) that is preheated over medium-high heat. Cook and stir until the sauce reduces by about a third.
5. Add the fried turkey thighs to the wok; gently stir to coat with the sauce.
6. Let the turkey rest for 10 minutes before slicing and serving. Enjoy!

258.Lime And Thyme Duck

Servings: 4
Cooking Time: 17 Minutes
Ingredients:
- 1-pound duck breast, skinless, boneless
- 2 oz preserved lime, sliced
- 1 teaspoon apple cider vinegar
- 1 tablespoon olive oil
- ½ teaspoon salt
- ½ teaspoon dried thyme

Directions:
1. Cut the duck breast on 4 pieces and sprinkle with salt, dried thyme, apple cider vinegar, and oil. Mix up the duck pieces well and put

on the foil. Then pot the reserved lime over the duck and wrap the foil. Preheat the air fryer to 375F and put the wrapped duck breast in the air fryer basket. Cook it for 17 minutes.

259.Cornish Game Hens

Servings:4
Cooking Time:16 Minutes
Ingredients:
- 1 teaspoon fresh rosemary, chopped
- 1 teaspoon fresh thyme, chopped
- 2 pounds Cornish game hen, backbone removed and halved
- ½ cup olive oil
- ¼ teaspoon sugar
- ¼ teaspoon red pepper flakes, crushed
- Salt and black pepper, to taste
- 1 teaspoon fresh lemon zest, finely grated

Directions:
1. Preheat the Air fryer to 390 °F and grease an Air fryer basket.
2. Mix olive oil, herbs, lemon zest, sugar, and spices in a bowl.
3. Stir in the Cornish game hen and refrigerate to marinate well for about 24 hours.
4. Transfer the Cornish game hen to the Air fryer and cook for about 16 minutes.
5. Dish out the hen portions onto serving plates and serve hot.

260.Turkey With Cabbage

Servings: 4
Cooking Time: 25 Minutes
Ingredients:
- 1 pound turkey meat, ground
- A pinch of salt and black pepper
- 2 tablespoons butter, melted
- 1 ounce chicken stock
- 1 small red cabbage head, shredded
- 1 tablespoon sweet paprika, chopped
- 1 tablespoon parsley, chopped

Directions:
1. Heat up a pan that fits the air fryer with the butter, add the meat and brown for 5 minutes. Add all the other ingredients, toss, put the pan in the air fryer and cook at 380 degrees F for 20 minutes. Divide everything between plates and serve.

261.Chicken, Mushrooms And Peppers Pan

Servings: 5
Cooking Time: 22 Minutes
Ingredients:
- 1-pound chicken breast, skinless, boneless
- 1 teaspoon minced ginger
- ½ teaspoon minced garlic
- 1 tablespoon coconut aminos

- 1 teaspoon lemon juice
- 5 oz cremini mushrooms, sliced
- ¼ cup bell pepper, sliced
- 5 oz cauliflower, chopped
- 1 teaspoon ground paprika
- ½ teaspoon cayenne pepper
- 1 tablespoon avocado oil
- 1 teaspoon salt

Directions:
1. Preheat the air fryer to 375F. In the mixing bowl mix up sliced mushrooms, cauliflower, and bell pepper. Sprinkle the ingredients with salt, ½ tablespoon avocado oil, cayenne pepper, and ground paprika. Mix up the vegetables and place them in the air fryer basket. Cook the ingredients for 5 minutes. Then shake them well and cook for 3 minutes more. Transfer the cooked vegetables into the bowl. Then preheat the air fryer to 380F. Slice the chicken breast into the strips. Sprinkle the sliced chicken breast with minced ginger, minced garlic, and sprinkle with coconut aminos and lemon juice. Place the chicken breast in the air fryer and cook it for 13 minutes. Then add cooked vegetables and mix up the meal. Cook it for 1 minute more.

262.Crispy Chicken Tenders With Hot Aioli

Servings:4
Cooking Time: 15 Minutes
Ingredients:
- 4 tbsp olive oil
- 1 cup breadcrumbs
- Salt and pepper to taste
- ½ tbsp garlic powder
- ½ tbsp ground chili
- Aioli:
- ½ cup mayonnaise
- 2 tbsp olive oil
- ½ tbsp ground chili

Directions:
1. Mix breadcrumbs, salt, pepper, garlic powder and chili, and spread onto a plate. Spray the chicken with oil. Roll the strips in the breadcrumb mixture until well coated. Spray with a little bit of oil.
2. Arrange an even layer of strips into your air fryer and cook for 6 minutes at 360 F, turning once halfway through. To prepare the hot aioli: combine mayo with oil and ground chili. Serve hot.

263.Middle Eastern Chicken Bbq With Tzatziki Sauce

Servings:6
Cooking Time: 24 Minutes
Ingredients:

- 1 1/2 pounds skinless, boneless chicken breast halves - cut into bite-sized pieces
- 1 teaspoon dried oregano
- 1/2 teaspoon salt
- 1/4 cup olive oil
- 2 cloves garlic, minced
- 2 tablespoons lemon juice
- Tzatziki Dip Ingredients
- 1 (6 ounce) container plain Greek-style yogurt
- 1 tablespoon olive oil
- 2 teaspoons white vinegar
- 1 clove garlic, minced
- 1 pinch salt
- 1/2 cucumber - peeled, seeded, and grated

Directions:
1. In a medium bowl mix well, all Tzatziki dip Ingredients. Refrigerate for at least 2 hours to allow flavors to blend.
2. In a resealable bag, mix well salt, oregano, garlic, lemon juice, and olive oil. Add chicken, squeeze excess air, seal, and marinate for at least 2 hours.
3. Thread chicken into skewers and place on skewer rack. Cook in batches.
4. For 12 minutes, cook on 360 °F. Halfway through cooking time, turnover skewers and baste with marinade from resealable bag.
5. Serve and enjoy with Tzatziki dip.

264. Kung Pao Chicken

Servings: 4
Cooking Time: 50 Minutes
Ingredients:
- 1 ½ pounds chicken breast, halved
- 1 tablespoon lemon juice
- 2 tablespoons mirin
- 1/4 cup milk
- 2 tablespoons soy sauce
- 1 tablespoon olive oil
- 1 teaspoon ginger, peeled and grated
- 2 garlic cloves, minced
- 1/2 teaspoon salt
- 1/2 teaspoon Szechuan pepper
- 1/2 teaspoon xanthan gum

Directions:
1. In a large ceramic dish, place the chicken, lemon juice, mirin, milk, soy sauce, olive oil, ginger, and garlic. Let it marinate for 30 minutes in your refrigerator.
2. Spritz the sides and bottom of the cooking basket with a nonstick cooking spray. Arrange the chicken in the cooking basket and cook at 370 degrees F for 10 minutes.
3. Turn over the chicken, baste with the reserved marinade and cook for 4 minutes longer. Taste for doneness, season with salt and pepper, and reserve.

4. Add the marinade to the preheated skillet over medium heat; add in xanthan gum. Let it cook for 5 to 6 minutes until the sauce thickens.
5. Spoon the sauce over the reserved chicken and serve immediately.

265. Chicken Gruyere

Servings: 4
Cooking Time: 20 Minutes
Ingredients:
- ¼ cup Gruyere cheese, grated
- 1 pound chicken breasts, boneless, skinless
- ½ cup flour
- 2 eggs, beaten
- Sea salt and black pepper to taste
- 4 lemon slices

Directions:
1. Preheat your Air Fryer to 370 F. Spray the air fryer basket with cooking spray.
2. Mix the breadcrumbs with Gruyere cheese in a bowl, pour the eggs in another bowl, and the flour in a third bowl. Toss the chicken in the flour, then in the eggs, and then in the breadcrumb mixture. Place in the fryer basket, close and cook for 12 minutes. At the 6-minute mark, turn the chicken over. Once golden brown, remove onto a serving plate and serve topped with lemon slices.

266. Savory Chives 'n Bacon Frittata

Servings: 4
Cooking Time: 15 Minutes
Ingredients:
- 1 tablespoon chives
- 6 eggs, beaten
- 6 uncured bacon, fried and crumbled
- Salt and pepper to taste

Directions:
1. Preheat the air fryer for 5 minutes.
2. Mix all ingredients in a mixing bowl.
3. Pour the mixture in a greased baking dish that will fit in the air fryer.
4. Close and cook for 15 minutes at 350°F.

267. Yogurt Chicken Thighs

Servings: 4
Cooking Time: 20 Minutes
Ingredients:
- 4 chicken thighs, skinless, boneless
- 2 tablespoons plain yogurt
- 1 teaspoon cayenne pepper
- 1 teaspoon dried cilantro
- ½ teaspoon ground cloves
- 1 tablespoon apple cider vinegar
- 1 teaspoon olive oil

Directions:

1. Make the marinade: in the mixing bowl mix up plain yogurt, cayenne pepper, dried cilantro, ground cloves, and apple cider vinegar. Then put the chicken thighs in the marinade and mix up well. Marinate the chicken for 20 minutes in the fridge. Then preheat the air fryer to 380F. Sprinkle the chicken thighs with olive oil and place in the air fryer. Cook them for 20 minutes.

268.Traditional Chicken Teriyaki

Servings: 4
Cooking Time: 50 Minutes
Ingredients:
- 1 ½ pounds chicken breast, halved
- 1 tablespoon lemon juice
- 2 tablespoons Mirin
- 1/4 cup milk
- 2 tablespoons soy sauce
- 1 tablespoon olive oil
- 1 teaspoon ginger, peeled and grated
- 2 garlic cloves, minced
- 1/2 teaspoon salt
- 1/2 teaspoon ground black pepper
- 1 teaspoon cornstarch

Directions:
1. In a large ceramic dish, place the chicken, lemon juice, Mirin, milk, soy sauce, olive oil, ginger, and garlic. Let it marinate for 30 minutes in your refrigerator.
2. Spritz the sides and bottom of the cooking basket with a nonstick cooking spray. Arrange the chicken in the cooking basket and cook at 370 degrees F for 10 minutes.
3. Turn over the chicken, baste with the reserved marinade and cook for 4 minutes longer. Taste for doneness, season with salt and pepper, and reserve.
4. Mix the cornstarch with 1 tablespoon of water. Add the marinade to the preheated skillet over medium heat; cook for 3 to 4 minutes. Now, stir in the cornstarch slurry and cook until the sauce thickens.
5. Spoon the sauce over the reserved chicken and serve immediately.

269.Marjoram Chicken

Servings: 2
Cooking Time: 1 Hr.
Ingredients:
- 2 skinless, boneless small chicken breasts
- 2 tbsp. butter
- 1 tsp. sea salt
- ½ tsp. red pepper flakes, crushed
- 2 tsp. marjoram
- ¼ tsp. lemon pepper

Directions:

1. In a bowl, coat the chicken breasts with all of the other ingredients. Set aside to marinate for 30 – 60 minutes.
2. Pre-heat your Air Fryer to 390 degrees.
3. Cook for 20 minutes, turning halfway through cooking time.
4. Check for doneness using an instant-read thermometer. Serve over jasmine rice.

270.Crispy Chicken Tenders

Servings:3
Cooking Time: 30 Minutes
Ingredients:
- 2 (6-ounces) boneless, skinless chicken breasts, pounded into ½-inch thickness and cut into tenders
- ¾ cup buttermilk
- 1½ teaspoons Worcestershire sauce, divided
- ½ teaspoon smoked paprika, divided
- Salt and ground black pepper, as required
- ½ cup all-purpose flour
- 1½ cups panko breadcrumbs
- ¼ cup Parmesan cheese, finely grated
- 2 tablespoons butter, melted
- 2 large eggs

Directions:
1. In a large bowl, mix together buttermilk, ¾ teaspoon of Worcestershire sauce, ¼ teaspoon of paprika, salt, and black pepper.
2. Add in the chicken tenders and refrigerate overnight.
3. In another bowl, mix together the flour, remaining paprika, salt, and black pepper.
4. Place the remaining Worcestershire sauce and eggs in a third bowl and beat until well combined.
5. Mix well the panko, Parmesan, and butter in a fourth bowl.
6. Remove the chicken tenders from bowl and discard the buttermilk.
7. Coat the chicken tenders with flour mixture, then dip into egg mixture and finally coat with the panko mixture.
8. Set the temperature of air fryer to 400 degrees F. Grease an air fryer basket.
9. Arrange chicken tenders into the prepared air fryer basket in 2 batches in a single layer.
10. Air fry for about 13-15 minutes, flipping once halfway through.
11. Remove from air fryer and transfer the chicken tenders onto a serving platter.
12. Serve hot.

271.Herbed Turkey Breast

Servings:3
Cooking Time:35 Minutes
Ingredients:

- 1 (2½-pounds) bone-in, skin-on turkey breast
- 1 teaspoon dried thyme, crushed
- 1 teaspoon dried rosemary, crushed
- ½ teaspoon dried sage, crushed
- ½ teaspoon dark brown sugar
- ½ teaspoon garlic powder
- ½ teaspoon paprika
- 1 tablespoon olive oil

Directions:
1. Preheat the Air fryer to 360 °F and grease an Air fryer basket.
2. Mix the herbs, brown sugar, and spices in a bowl.
3. Drizzle the turkey breast with oil and season with the herb mixture.
4. Arrange the turkey breast into the Air Fryer basket, skin side down and cook for about 35 minutes, flipping once in between.
5. Dish out in a platter and cut into desired size slices to serve.

272.Crispy & Juicy Whole Chicken

Servings: 8
Cooking Time: 60 Minutes
Ingredients:
- 5 lbs chicken, wash and remove giblets
- 1/2 tsp onion powder
- 1/2 tsp pepper
- 1 tsp paprika
- 1 tsp dried oregano
- 1 tsp dried basil
- 1 1/2 tsp salt

Directions:
1. Preheat the air fryer to 360 F.
2. Mix together all spices and rub over chicken.
3. Place chicken into the air fryer basket. Make sure the chicken breast side down.
4. Cook chicken for 30 minutes then turn to another side and cook for 30 minutes more.
5. Slice and serve.

273.Oregano And Lemon Chicken Drumsticks

Servings: 4
Cooking Time: 21 Minutes
Ingredients:
- 4 chicken drumsticks, with skin, bone-in
- 1 teaspoon dried cilantro
- ½ teaspoon dried oregano
- ½ teaspoon salt
- 1 teaspoon lemon juice
- 1 teaspoon butter, softened
- 2 garlic cloves, diced

Directions:
1. In the mixing bowl mix up dried cilantro, oregano, and salt. Then fill the chicken drumstick's skin with a cilantro mixture. Add butter and diced garlic. Sprinkle the

chicken with lemon juice. Preheat the air fryer to 375F. Put the chicken drumsticks in the air fryer and cook them for 21 minutes.

274.Duck Breasts And Mango Mix Recipe

Servings: 4
Cooking Time:1 Hour 10 Minutes
Ingredients:
- 4 duck breasts
- 3 garlic cloves; minced
- 2 tbsp. olive oil
- 1½ tbsp. lemongrass; chopped.
- 3 tbsp. lemon juice
- Salt and black pepper to the taste
- For the mango mix:
- 1 mango; peeled and chopped
- 1 ½ tbsp. lemon juice
- 1 tbsp. coriander; chopped
- 1 red onion; chopped
- 1 tsp. ginger; grated
- 3/4 tsp. sugar
- 1 tbsp. sweet chili sauce

Directions:
1. In a bowl, mix duck breasts with salt, pepper, lemongrass, 3 tbsp. lemon juice, olive oil and garlic; toss well, keep in the fridge for 1 hour, transfer to your air fryer and cook at 360 °F, for 10 minutes; flipping once.
2. Meanwhile; in a bowl, mix mango with coriander, onion, chili sauce, lemon juice, ginger and sugar and toss well.
3. Divide duck on plates, add mango mix on the side and serve.

275.Gingered Chicken Drumsticks

Servings:3
Cooking Time:25 Minutes
Ingredients:
- ¼ cup full-fat coconut milk
- 3 (6-ounces) chicken drumsticks
- 2 teaspoons fresh ginger, minced
- 2 teaspoons galangal, minced
- 2 teaspoons ground turmeric
- Salt, to taste

Directions:
1. Preheat the Air fryer to 375 °F and grease an Air fryer basket.
2. Mix the coconut milk, galangal, ginger, and spices in a bowl.
3. Add the chicken drumsticks and coat generously with the marinade.
4. Refrigerate to marinate for at least 8 hours and transfer into the Air fryer basket.
5. Cook for about 25 minutes and dish out the chicken drumsticks onto a serving platter.

276.Vermouth Bacon And Turkey Burgers

Servings: 4

Cooking Time: 30 Minutes
Ingredients:
- 2 tablespoons vermouth
- 1 tablespoon honey
- 2 strips Canadian bacon, sliced
- 1 pound ground turkey
- 1/2 shallot, minced
- 2 garlic cloves, minced
- 2 tablespoons fish sauce
- Sea salt and ground black pepper, to taste
- 1 teaspoon red pepper flakes
- 4 soft hamburger rolls
- 4 tablespoons tomato ketchup
- 4 tablespoons mayonnaise
- 4 (1-ounce slices Cheddar cheese
- 4 lettuce leaves

Directions:
1. Start by preheating your Air Fryer to 400 degrees F.
2. Whisk the vermouth and honey in a mixing bowl; brush the Canadian bacon with the vermouth mixture.
3. Cook for 3 minutes. Flip the bacon over and cook an additional 3 minutes.
4. Then, thoroughly combine the ground turkey, shallots, garlic, fish sauce, salt, black pepper, and red pepper. Form the meat mixture into 4 burger patties.
5. Bake in the preheated Air Fryer at 370 degrees F for 10 minutes. Flip them over and cook another 10 minutes.
6. Spread the ketchup and mayonnaise on the inside of the hamburger rolls and place the burgers on the rolls; top with bacon, cheese and lettuce; serve immediately.

277.Spicy Asian Chicken Thighs

Servings: 4
Cooking Time: 20 Minutes
Ingredients:
- 4 chicken thighs, skin-on, and bone-in
- 2 tsp ginger, grated
- 1 lime juice
- 2 tbsp chili garlic sauce
- 1/4 cup olive oil
- 1/3 cup soy sauce

Directions:
1. In a large bowl, whisk together ginger, lime juice, chili garlic sauce, oil, and soy sauce.
2. Add chicken in bowl and coat well with marinade and place in the refrigerator for 30 minutes.
3. Place marinated chicken in air fryer basket and cook at 400 F for 15-20 minutes or until the internal temperature of chicken reaches at 165 F. Turn chicken halfway through.
4. Serve and enjoy.

278.Paprika Duck

Servings: 6
Cooking Time: 28 Minutes
Ingredients:
- 10 oz duck skin
- 1 teaspoon sunflower oil
- ½ teaspoon salt
- ½ teaspoon ground paprika

Directions:
1. Preheat the air fryer to 375F. Then sprinkle the duck skin with sunflower oil, salt, and ground paprika. Put the duck skin in the air fryer and cook it for 18 minutes. Then flip it on another side and cook for 10 minutes more or until it is crunchy from both sides.

279.Mediterranean-style Duck With Gravy

Servings: 4
Cooking Time: 25 Minutes
Ingredients:
- 1 ½ pounds smoked duck breasts, boneless
- 1 tablespoon yellow mustard
- 2 tablespoons ketchup, low-carb
- 8 pearl onions peeled
- 5 ounces chicken broth
- 2 egg yolks, whisked
- 1 teaspoon rosemary, finely chopped

Directions:
1. Cook the smoked duck breasts in the preheated Air Fryer at 365 degrees F for 15 minutes.
2. Smear the mustard and ketchup on the duck breast. Top with pearl onions. Cook for a further 7 minutes or until the skin of the duck breast looks crispy and golden brown.
3. Slice the duck breasts and reserve. Drain off the duck fat from the pan.
4. Then, add the reserved 1 tablespoon of duck fat to the pan and warm it over medium heat; add chicken broth and bring to a boil.
5. Gently fold in the whisked egg yolks and rosemary. Reduce the heat to low and cook until the gravy has thickened slightly. Spoon the warm gravy over the reserved duck breasts. Enjoy!

280.Simple Paprika Duck

Servings: 4
Cooking Time: 25 Minutes
Ingredients:
- 1 pound duck breasts, skinless, boneless and cubed
- Salt and black pepper to the taste
- 1 tablespoon olive oil
- ½ teaspoon sweet paprika
- ¼ cup chicken stock
- 1 teaspoon thyme, chopped

Directions:

1. Heat up a pan that fits your air fryer with the oil over medium heat, add the duck pieces, and brown them for 5 minutes. Add the rest of the ingredients, toss, put the pan in the machine and cook at 380 degrees F for 20 minutes. Divide between plates and serve.

281.Tomato Chicken Mix

Servings: 4
Cooking Time: 18 Minutes
Ingredients:
- 1-pound chicken breast, skinless, boneless
- 1 tablespoon keto tomato sauce
- 1 teaspoon avocado oil
- ½ teaspoon garlic powder

Directions:
1. In the small bowl mix up tomato sauce, avocado oil, and garlic powder. Then brush the chicken breast with the tomato sauce mixture well. Preheat the air fryer to 385F. Place the chicken breast in the air fryer and cook it for 15 minutes. Then flip it on another side and cook for 3 minutes more. Slice the cooked chicken breast into servings.

282.Duck Breast With Figs

Servings:2
Cooking Time:45 Minutes
Ingredients:
- 1 pound boneless duck breast
- 6 fresh figs, halved
- 1 tablespoon fresh thyme, chopped
- 2 cups fresh pomegranate juice
- 2 tablespoons lemon juice
- 3 tablespoons brown sugar
- 1 teaspoon olive oil
- Salt and black pepper, as required

Directions:
1. Preheat the Air fryer to 400 °F and grease an Air fryer basket.
2. Put the pomegranate juice, lemon juice, and brown sugar in a medium saucepan over medium heat.
3. Bring to a boil and simmer on low heat for about 25 minutes.
4. Season the duck breasts generously with salt and black pepper.
5. Arrange the duck breasts into the Air fryer basket, skin side up and cook for about 14 minutes, flipping once in between.
6. Dish out the duck breasts onto a cutting board for about 10 minutes.
7. Meanwhile, put the figs, olive oil, salt, and black pepper in a bowl until well mixed.
8. Set the Air fryer to 400 °F and arrange the figs into the Air fryer basket.

9. Cook for about 5 more minutes and dish out in a platter.
10. Put the duck breast with the roasted figs and drizzle with warm pomegranate juice mixture.
11. Garnish with fresh thyme and serve warm.

283.Sweet Sriracha Turkey Legs

Servings:2
Cooking Time:35 Minutes
Ingredients:
- 1-pound turkey legs
- 1 tablespoon butter
- 1 tablespoon cilantro
- 1 tablespoon chives
- 1 tablespoon scallions
- 4 tablespoons sriracha sauce
- 1½ tablespoons soy sauce
- ½ lime, juiced

Directions:
1. Preheat the Air fryer on Roasting mode to 360 °F for 3 minutes and grease an Air fryer basket.
2. Arrange the turkey legs in the Air fryer basket and cook for about 30 minutes, flipping several times in between.
3. Mix butter, scallions, sriracha sauce, soy sauce and lime juice in the saucepan and cook for about for 3 minutes until the sauce thickens.
4. Drizzle this sauce over the turkey legs and garnish with cilantro and chives to serve.

284.Creamy Chicken 'n Pasta Tetrazzini

Servings:3
Cooking Time: 30 Minutes
Ingredients:
- 1 cup chopped cooked chicken breast
- 1/2 (10.75 ounce) can condensed cream of mushroom soup
- 1/2 cup chicken broth
- 1/2 cup shredded sharp Cheddar cheese
- 1/4 (10 ounce) package frozen green peas
- 1/4 cup grated Parmesan cheese
- 1/4 cup minced green bell pepper
- 1/4 cup minced onion
- 1/4 teaspoon salt
- 1/4 teaspoon Worcestershire sauce
- 1/8 teaspoon ground black pepper
- 2 tablespoons butter
- 2 tablespoons cooking sherry
- 3/4 cup sliced fresh mushrooms
- 4-ounce linguine pasta, cooked following manufacturer's Directions:

Directions:
1. Lightly grease baking pan of air fryer and melt butter for 2 minutes at 360 °F. Stir in bell pepper, onion, and mushrooms. Cook for 5 minutes.

2. Add chicken broth and mushroom soup, mix well. Cook for 5 minutes.
3. Mix in chicken, pepper, salt, Worcestershire sauce, sherry, peas, cheddar cheese, and pasta. Sprinkle paprika and Parmesan on top.
4. Cook for 15 minutes at 390 °F until tops are lightly browned.
5. Serve and enjoy.

285. Chicken-veggie Fusilli Casserole

Servings:3
Cooking Time: 30 Minutes
Ingredients:
- 1 cup frozen mixed vegetables
- 1 tablespoon butter, melted
- 1 tablespoon grated Parmesan cheese
- 1 tablespoon olive oil
- 1/2 (10.75 ounce) can condensed cream of chicken soup
- 1/2 (10.75 ounce) can condensed cream of mushroom soup
- 1/2 cup dry bread crumbs
- 1/2 cup dry fusilli pasta, cooked according to manufacturer's Directions:
- 1-1/2 teaspoons dried basil
- 1-1/2 teaspoons dried minced onion
- 1-1/2 teaspoons dried parsley
- 3 chicken tenderloins, cut into chunks
- garlic powder to taste
- salt and pepper to taste

Directions:
1. Lightly grease baking pan of air fryer with olive oil. Add chicken. Season with parsley, basil, garlic powder, pepper, salt, and minced onion.
2. For 10 minutes, cook on 360 °F. Stir chicken halfway through cooking time.
3. Remove basket and toss the mixture a bit. Stir in mixed vegetables, cream of mushroom soup, cream of chicken soup, and cooked pasta. Mix well.
4. Mix melted butter, parmesan, and bread crumbs in a small bowl. Evenly spread on top of casserole.
5. Cook for 20 minutes at 390 °F.
6. Serve and enjoy.

286. Buffalo Chicken Wings

Servings: 3
Cooking Time: 37 Minutes
Ingredients:
- 2 lb. chicken wings
- 1 tsp. salt
- ¼ tsp. black pepper
- 1 cup buffalo sauce

Directions:
1. Wash the chicken wings and pat them dry with clean kitchen towels.

2. Place the chicken wings in a large bowl and sprinkle on salt and pepper.
3. Pre-heat the Air Fryer to 380°F.
4. Place the wings in the fryer and cook for 15 minutes, giving them an occasional stir throughout.
5. Place the wings in a bowl. Pour over the buffalo sauce and toss well to coat.
6. Put the chicken back in the Air Fryer and cook for a final 5 – 6 minutes.

287. Simple Spice Chicken Wings

Servings: 3
Cooking Time: 30 Minutes
Ingredients:
- 1 1/2 lbs chicken wings
- 1 tbsp baking powder, gluten-free
- 1/2 tsp onion powder
- 1/2 tsp garlic powder
- 1/2 tsp smoked paprika
- 1 tbsp olive oil
- 1/2 tsp pepper
- 1/4 tsp sea salt

Directions:
1. Add chicken wings and oil in a large mixing bowl and toss well.
2. Mix together remaining ingredients and sprinkle over chicken wings and toss to coat.
3. Spray air fryer basket with cooking spray.
4. Add chicken wings in air fryer basket and cook at 400 F for 15 minutes. Toss well.
5. Turn chicken wings to another side and cook for 15 minutes more.
6. Serve and enjoy.

288. Balsamic Ginger Duck

Servings: 4
Cooking Time: 30 Minutes
Ingredients:
- 12 oz duck legs
- 1 tablespoon balsamic vinegar
- 1 teaspoon Splenda
- ½ teaspoon minced ginger
- ½ teaspoon harissa
- 1 tablespoon avocado oil

Directions:
1. Rub the duck legs with minced ginger, harissa, Splenda, and avocado oil. Then sprinkle the duck legs with ½ tablespoon of balsamic vinegar. Preheat the air fryer to 385F. Place the duck legs in the air fryer and cook them for 30 minutes. Sprinkle the cooked duck legs with the balsamic vinegar and place it in the serving plates.

289. The Best Chicken Burgers Ever

Servings: 4
Cooking Time: 20 Minutes
Ingredients:

- 1 tablespoon olive oil
- 1 onion, peeled and finely chopped
- 2 garlic cloves, minced
- Sea salt and ground black pepper, to taste
- 1/2 teaspoon paprika
- 1/2 teaspoon ground cumin
- 1 pound chicken breast, ground
- 4 soft rolls
- 4 tablespoons ketchup
- 4 tablespoons mayonnaise
- 2 teaspoons Dijon mustard
- 4 tablespoons green onions, chopped
- 4 pickles, sliced

Directions:
1. Heat the olive oil in a skillet over high flame. Then, sauté the onion until golden and translucent, about 4 minutes.
2. Add the garlic and cook an additional 30 seconds or until it is aromatic. Season with salt, pepper, paprika, and cumin; reserve.
3. Add the chicken and cook for 2 to 3 minutes, stirring and crumbling with a fork. Add the onion mixture and mix to combine well.
4. Shape the mixture into patties and transfer them to the cooking basket. Cook in the preheated Air Fryer at 360 degrees F for 6 minutes. Turn them over and cook an additional 5 minutes. Work in batches.
5. Smear the base of the roll with ketchup, mayo, and mustard. Top with the chicken, green onions, and pickles. Enjoy!

290.Bbq Turkey Meatballs With Cranberry Sauce

Servings:4
Cooking Time: 25 Minutes
Ingredients:
- 1 ½ tablespoons water
- 2 teaspoons cider vinegar
- 1 tsp salt and more to taste
- 1-pound ground turkey
- 1 1/2 tablespoons barbecue sauce
- 1/3 cup cranberry sauce
- 1/4-pound ground bacon

Directions:
1. In a bowl, mix well with hands the turkey, ground bacon and a tsp of salt. Evenly form into 16 equal sized balls.
2. In a small saucepan boil cranberry sauce, barbecue sauce, water, cider vinegar, and a dash or two of salt. Mix well and simmer for 3 minutes.
3. Thread meatballs in skewers and baste with cranberry sauce. Place on skewer rack in air fryer.
4. For 15 minutes, cook on 360 °F. Every after 5 minutes of cooking time, turnover skewers and baste with sauce. If needed, cook in batches.

5. Serve and enjoy.

291.Curried Drumsticks

Servings: 2
Cooking Time: 22 Minutes
Ingredients:
- 2 turkey drumsticks
- 1/3 cup coconut milk
- 1 1/2 tbsp ginger, minced
- 1/4 tsp cayenne pepper
- 2 tbsp red curry paste
- 1/4 tsp pepper
- 1 tsp kosher salt

Directions:
1. Add all ingredients into the bowl and stir to coat. Place in refrigerator for overnight.
2. Spray air fryer basket with cooking spray.
3. Place marinated drumsticks into the air fryer basket and cook at 390 F for 22 minutes.
4. Serve and enjoy.

292.Goulash

Servings: 2
Cooking Time: 20 Minutes
Ingredients:
- 2 chopped bell peppers
- 2 diced tomatoes
- 1 lb. ground chicken
- ½ cup chicken broth
- Salt and pepper

Directions:
1. Pre-heat your fryer at 365°F and spray with cooking spray.
2. Cook the bell pepper for five minutes.
3. Add in the diced tomatoes and ground chicken. Combine well, then allow to cook for a further six minutes.
4. Pour in chicken broth, and season to taste with salt and pepper. Cook for another six minutes before serving.

293.Asian Chicken Filets With Cheese

Servings: 2
Cooking Time: 50 Minutes
Ingredients:
- 4 rashers smoked bacon
- 2 chicken filets
- 1/2 teaspoon coarse sea salt
- 1/4 teaspoon black pepper, preferably freshly ground
- 1 teaspoon garlic, minced
- 1 (2-inch) piece ginger, peeled and minced
- 1 teaspoon black mustard seeds
- 1 teaspoon mild curry powder
- 1/2 cup coconut milk
- 1/3 cup tortilla chips, crushed
- 1/2 cup Pecorino Romano cheese, freshly grated

Directions:
1. Start by preheating your Air Fryer to 400 degrees F. Add the smoked bacon and cook in the preheated Air Fryer for 5 to 7 minutes. Reserve.
2. In a mixing bowl, place the chicken fillets, salt, black pepper, garlic, ginger, mustard seeds, curry powder, and milk. Let it marinate in your refrigerator about 30 minutes.
3. In another bowl, mix the crushed chips and grated Pecorino Romano cheese.
4. Dredge the chicken fillets through the chips mixture and transfer them to the cooking basket. Reduce the temperature to 380 degrees F and cook the chicken for 6 minutes.
5. Turn them over and cook for a further 6 minutes. Repeat the process until you have run out of ingredients.
6. Serve with reserved bacon. Enjoy!

294.Hot Chicken Wings

Servings: 4
Cooking Time: 30 Minutes
Ingredients:
- 1 tablespoon olive oil
- 2 pounds chicken wings
- 1 tablespoon lime juice
- 2 teaspoons smoked paprika
- 1 teaspoon red pepper flakes, crushed
- Salt and black pepper to the taste

Directions:
1. In a bowl, mix the chicken wings with all the other ingredients and toss well. Put the chicken wings in your air fryer's basket and cook at 380 degrees F for 15 minutes on each side. Divide between plates and serve with a side salad.

295.Ethiopian-style Chicken With Cauliflower

Servings: 6
Cooking Time: 30 Minutes
Ingredients:
- 2 handful fresh Italian parsleys, roughly chopped
- ½ cup fresh chopped chives
- 2 sprigs thyme
- 6 chicken drumsticks
- 1 ½ small-sized head cauliflower, broken into large-sized florets
- For the Berbere Spice Rub Mix:
- 2 teaspoons mustard powder
- 1/3 teaspoon porcini powder
- 1 ½ teaspoons berbere spice
- 1/3teaspoon sweet paprika
- 1/2 teaspoon shallot powder
- 1teaspoon granulated garlic

- 1 teaspoon freshly cracked pink peppercorns
- 1/2 teaspoon sea salt

Directions:
1. Simply combine all items for the berbere spice rub mix. After that, coat the chicken drumsticks with this rub mix on all sides. Transfer them to the baking dish.
2. Now, lower the cauliflower onto the chicken drumsticks. Add thyme, chives and Italian parsley and spritz everything with a pan spray. Transfer the baking dish to the preheated Air Fryer.
3. Next step, set the timer for 28 minutes; roast at 355 degrees F, turning occasionally. Bon appétit!

296.Oats Crusted Chicken Breasts

Servings:2
Cooking Time:12 Minutes
Ingredients:
- 2 (6-ounces) chicken breasts
- ¾ cup oats
- 1 tablespoon fresh parsley
- 2 medium eggs
- Salt and black pepper, to taste
- 2 tablespoons mustard powder

Directions:
1. Preheat the Air fryer to 350 °F and grease an Air fryer grill pan.
2. Season the chicken pieces with salt and black pepper and keep aside.
3. Put the oats, mustard powder, parsley, salt and black pepper in a blender and pulse until coarse.
4. Place the oat mixture into a shallow bowl and whisk the eggs in another bowl.
5. Dredge the chicken in the oat mixture and dip into the whisked eggs.
6. Arrange the chicken breasts into the Air fryer grill pan and cook for about 12 minutes, flipping once in between.
7. Dish out the chicken into a serving platter and serve hot.

297.Duck Rolls

Servings:3
Cooking Time:40 Minutes
Ingredients:
- 1 pound duck breast fillet, each cut into 2 pieces
- 3 tablespoons fresh parsley, finely chopped
- 1 small red onion, finely chopped
- 1 garlic clove, crushed
- 1½ teaspoons ground cumin
- 1 teaspoon ground cinnamon
- ½ teaspoon red chili powder
- Salt, to taste
- 2 tablespoons olive oil

Directions:
1. Preheat the Air fryer to 355 °F and grease an Air fryer basket.
2. Mix the garlic, parsley, onion, spices, and 1 tablespoon of olive oil in a bowl.
3. Make a slit in each duck piece horizontally and coat with onion mixture.
4. Roll each duck piece tightly and transfer into the Air fryer basket.
5. Cook for about 40 minutes and cut into desired size slices to serve.

298.Quick And Crispy Chicken

Servings:4
Cooking Time: 15 Minutes
Ingredients:
- 2 tbsp butter
- 2 oz breadcrumbs
- 1 large egg, whisked

Directions:
1. Preheat air fryer to 380 F. Combine butter the breadcrumbs in a bowl. Keep mixing and stirring until the mixture gets crumbly. Dip the chicken in the egg wash. Then dip the chicken in the crumbs mix. Cook for 10 minutes. Serve.

299.Sweet Chicken Breasts

Servings:2
Cooking Time: 35 Minutes
Ingredients:
- 1 tablespoon maple syrup
- 2 teaspoons minced fresh rosemary
- ¼ teaspoon salt
- ⅛ teaspoon black pepper
- 2 chicken breasts, boneless, skinless
- Cooking spray

Directions:
1. In a bowl, mix mustard, maple syrup, rosemary, salt, and pepper. Rub mixture onto chicken breasts. Spray generously the air fryer basket generously with cooking spray. Arrange the breasts inside and cook for 20 minutes, turning once halfway through.

300.Chinese Style Chicken

Servings:4
Cooking Time: 40 Minutes
Ingredients:
- 2 teaspoons brown sugar
- 1 ½ teaspoon five spice powder
- Salt and pepper to taste
- 2 chicken breasts, halved
- 3 ½ teaspoon grated ginger
- ¼ cup hoisin sauce
- 2 tablespoons rice vinegar
- 3 ½ teaspoons honey
- 1 ¼ teaspoons sesame oil

- 3 cucumbers, sliced

Directions:
1. Place all ingredients, except for the cucumber, in a Ziploc bag.
2. Allow to rest in the fridge for at least 2 hours.
3. Preheat the air fryer at 375°F.
4. Place the grill pan accessory in the air fryer.
5. Grill for 40 minutes and make sure to flip the chicken often for even cooking.
6. Serve chicken with cucumber once cooked.

301.Aromatic Turkey Breast With Mustard

Servings: 4
Cooking Time: 1 Hour
Ingredients:
- 1/2 teaspoon dried thyme
- 1 ½ pounds turkey breasts
- 1/2 teaspoon dried sage
- 3 whole star anise
- 1 ½ tablespoons olive oil
- 1 ½ tablespoons hot mustard
- 1 teaspoon smoked cayenne pepper
- 1 teaspoon fine sea salt

Directions:
1. Set your Air Fryer to cook at 365 degrees F.
2. Brush the turkey breast with olive oil and sprinkle with seasonings.
3. Cook at 365 degrees F for 45 minutes, turning twice. Now, pause the machine and spread the cooked breast with the hot mustard.
4. Air-fry for 6 to 8 more minutes. Let it rest before slicing and serving. Bon appétit!

302.Lemon Grilled Chicken Breasts

Servings:6
Cooking Time: 40 Minutes
Ingredients:
- 3 tablespoons fresh lemon juice
- 2 tablespoons olive oil
- 2 cloves of garlic, minced
- 6 boneless chicken breasts, halved
- Salt and pepper to taste

Directions:
1. Place all ingredients in a Ziploc bag
2. Allow to marinate for at least 2 hours in the fridge.
3. Preheat the air fryer at 375°F.
4. Place the grill pan accessory in the air fryer.
5. Grill for 40 minutes and make sure to flip the chicken every 10 minutes for even cooking.

303.Tarragon Turkey Tenderloins With Baby Potatoes

Servings: 6
Cooking Time: 50 Minutes

Ingredients:
- 2 pounds turkey tenderloins
- 2 teaspoons olive oil
- Salt and ground black pepper, to taste
- 1 teaspoon smoked paprika
- 2 tablespoons dry white wine
- 1 tablespoon fresh tarragon leaves, chopped
- 1 pound baby potatoes, rubbed

Directions:
1. Brush the turkey tenderloins with olive oil. Season with salt, black pepper, and paprika.
2. Afterwards, add the white wine and tarragon.
3. Cook the turkey tenderloins at 350 degrees F for 30 minutes, flipping them over halfway through. Let them rest for 5 to 9 minutes before slicing and serving.
4. After that, spritz the sides and bottom of the cooking basket with the remaining 1 teaspoon of olive oil.
5. Then, preheat your Air Fryer to 400 degrees F; cook the baby potatoes for 15 minutes. Serve with the turkey and enjoy!

304.Chicken Legs

Servings: 4
Cooking Time: 35 Minutes
Ingredients:
- 3 chicken legs, bone-in, with ski
- 3 chicken thighs, bone-in, with skin
- 2 cups flour
- 1 cup buttermilk
- 1 tsp. salt
- 1 tsp. ground black pepper
- 1 tsp. garlic powder
- 1 tsp. onion powder
- 1 tsp. ground cumin
- 2 tbsp. extra virgin olive oil

Directions:
1. Wash the chicken, dry it, and place it in a large bowl.

2. Pour the buttermilk over the chicken and refrigerate for 2 hours.
3. In a separate bowl, combine the flour with all of the seasonings.
4. Dip the chicken into the flour mixture. Dredge it the buttermilk before rolling it in the flour again.
5. Pre-heat the Air Fryer to 360°F
6. Put the chicken legs and thighs in the fryer basket. Drizzle on the olive oil and cook for roughly 20 minutes, flipping each piece of chicken a few times throughout the cooking time, until cooked through and crisped up.

305.Battered Chicken Thighs

Servings: 4
Cooking Time: 4 Hours 45 Minutes
Ingredients:
- 2 cups buttermilk
- 3 tsp. salt
- 1 tsp. cayenne pepper
- 1 tbsp. paprika
- 1 ½ lb. chicken thighs
- 2 tsp. black pepper
- 2 cups flour
- 1 tbsp. garlic powder
- 1 tbsp. baking powder

Directions:
1. Put the chicken thighs in a large bowl.
2. In a separate bowl, combine the buttermilk, salt, cayenne, and black pepper.
3. Coat the thighs with the buttermilk mixture. Place a sheet of aluminum foil over the bowl and set in the refrigerator for 4 hours.
4. Pre-heat your Air Fryer to 400°F.
5. Combine together the flour, baking powder, and paprika in a shallow bowl. Cover a baking dish with a layer of parchment paper.
6. Coat the chicken thighs in the flour mixture and bake in the fryer for 10 minutes. Turn the thighs over and air fry for another 8 minutes. You will have to do this in two batches.

BEEF,PORK & LAMB RECIPES

306.Simple Lamb Chops

Servings:2
Cooking Time:6 Minutes
Ingredients:
- 4 (4-ounces) lamb chops
- Salt and black pepper, to taste
- 1 tablespoon olive oil

Directions:
1. Preheat the Air fryer to 390 °F and grease an Air fryer basket.
2. Mix the olive oil, salt, and black pepper in a large bowl and add chops.
3. Arrange the chops in the Air fryer basket and cook for about 6 minutes.
4. Dish out the lamb chops and serve hot.

307.Pork Chops And Mushrooms Mix Recipe

Servings: 3
Cooking Time:50 Minutes
Ingredients:
- 8 oz. mushrooms; sliced
- 3 pork chops; boneless
- 1 tsp. nutmeg
- 1 tbsp. balsamic vinegar
- 1 tsp. garlic powder
- 1 yellow onion; chopped.
- 1 cup mayonnaise
- 1/2 cup olive oil

Directions:
1. Heat up a pan that fits your air fryer with the oil over medium heat, add mushrooms and onions; stir and cook for 4 minutes.
2. Add pork chops, nutmeg and garlic powder and brown on both sides.
3. Introduce pan your air fryer at 330 °F and cook for 30 minutes. Add vinegar and mayo; stir, divide everything on plates and serve.

308.Pork Chops And Roasted Peppers Recipe

Servings: 4
Cooking Time:26 Minutes
Ingredients:
- 3 tbsp. lemon juice
- 1 tbsp. smoked paprika
- 2 roasted bell peppers; chopped.
- 2 tbsp. thyme; chopped
- 3 garlic cloves; minced
- 3 tbsp. olive oil
- 4 pork chops; bone in
- Salt and black pepper to the taste

Directions:
1. In a pan that fits your air fryer, mix pork chops with oil, lemon juice, smoked paprika, thyme, garlic, bell peppers, salt and pepper, toss well, introduce in your air fryer and cook at 400 °F, for 16 minutes
2. Divide pork chops and peppers mix on plates and serve right away.

309.Beef & Broccoli

Servings: 4
Cooking Time: 25 Minutes
Ingredients:
- 1 lb. broccoli, cut into florets
- ¾ lb. round steak, cut into strips
- 1 garlic clove, minced
- 1 tsp. ginger, minced
- 1 tbsp. olive oil
- 1 tsp. cornstarch
- 1 tsp. sugar
- 1 tsp. soy sauce
- ⅓ cup sherry wine
- 2 tsp. sesame oil
- ⅓ cup oyster sauce

Directions:
1. In a bowl, combine the sugar, soy sauce, sherry wine, cornstarch, sesame oil, and oyster sauce.
2. Place the steak strips in the bowl, coat each one with the mixture and allow to marinate for 45 minutes.
3. Put the broccoli in the Air Fryer and lay the steak on top.
4. Top with the olive oil, garlic and ginger.
5. Cook at 350°F for 12 minutes. Serve hot with rice if desired.

310.Smoked Beef Roast

Servings: 8
Cooking Time: 45 Minutes
Ingredients:
- 2 lb. roast beef, at room temperature
- 2 tbsp. extra-virgin olive oil
- 1 tsp. sea salt flakes
- 1 tsp. black pepper, preferably freshly ground
- 1 tsp. smoked paprika
- Few dashes of liquid smoke
- 2 jalapeño peppers, thinly sliced

Directions:
1. Pre-heat the Air Fryer to 330°F.
2. With kitchen towels, pat the beef dry.
3. Massage the extra-virgin olive oil and seasonings into the meat. Cover with liquid smoke.
4. Place the beef in the Air Fryer and roast for 30 minutes. Flip the roast over and allow to cook for another 15 minutes.
5. When cooked through, serve topped with sliced jalapeños.

311.Pork Chops Crusted In Parmesan-paprika

Servings:6
Cooking Time: 35 Minutes
Ingredients:
- ¼ teaspoon pepper
- ½ teaspoon chili powder
- ½ teaspoon onion powder
- ½ teaspoon salt
- 1 cup pork rind crumbs
- 1 teaspoon smoked paprika
- 2 large eggs, beaten
- 3 tablespoons parmesan cheese
- 6 thick pork chops

Directions:
1. Season the pork chops with salt, pepper, paprika, onion, and chili powder. Allow to marinate in the fridge for at least 3 hours.
2. In a bowl, place the beaten egg.
3. In another bowl, combine the pork rind and parmesan cheese.
4. Preheat the air fryer to 390°F.
5. Dip the pork in beaten egg before dredging in the pork rind crumb mixture.
6. Place in the air fryer basket and cook for 30 to 35 minutes.

312.Ground Beef On Deep Dish Pizza

Servings:4
Cooking Time: 25 Minutes
Ingredients:
- 1 can (10-3/4 ounces) condensed tomato soup, undiluted
- 1 can (8 ounces) mushroom stems and pieces, drained
- 1 cup shredded part-skim mozzarella cheese
- 1 cup warm water (110°F to 115°F)
- 1 package (1/4 ounce) active dry yeast
- 1 small green pepper, julienned
- 1 teaspoon dried rosemary, crushed
- 1 teaspoon each dried basil, oregano and thyme
- 1 teaspoon salt
- 1 teaspoon sugar
- 1/4 teaspoon garlic powder
- 1-pound ground beef, cooked and drained
- 2 tablespoons canola oil
- 2-1/2 cups all-purpose flour

Directions:
1. In a large bowl, dissolve yeast in warm water. Add the sugar, salt, oil and 2 cups flour. Beat until smooth. Stir in enough remaining flour to form a soft dough. Cover and let rest for 20 minutes. Divide into two and store half in the freezer for future use.
2. On a floured surface, roll into a square the size of your air fryer. Transfer to a greased air fryer baking pan. Sprinkle with beef.
3. Mix well seasonings and soup in a small bowl and pour over beef.
4. Sprinkle top with mushrooms and green pepper. Top with cheese.
5. Cover pan with foil.
6. For 15 minutes, cook on 390 °F.
7. Remove foil, cook for another 10 minutes or until cheese is melted.
8. Serve and enjoy.

313.Ham And Veggie Air Fried Mix Recipe

Servings: 6
Cooking Time:30 Minutes
Ingredients:
- 1/4 cup butter
- 1/4 cup flour
- 6 oz. sweet peas
- 4 oz. mushrooms; halved
- 3 cups milk
- 1/2 tsp. thyme; dried
- 2 cups ham; chopped
- 1 cup baby carrots

Directions:
1. Heat up a large pan that fits your air fryer with the butter over medium heat, melt it, add flour and whisk well
2. Add milk and, well again and take off heat
3. Add thyme, ham, peas, mushrooms and baby carrots, toss, put in your air fryer and cook at 360 °F, for 20 minutes. Divide everything on plates and serve.

314.Stuffed Bell Pepper

Servings: 4
Cooking Time: 25 Minutes
Ingredients:
- 4 bell peppers, cut top of bell pepper
- 16 oz. ground beef
- 2/3 cup cheese, shredded
- ½ cup rice, cooked
- 1 tsp. basil, dried
- ½ tsp. chili powder
- 1 tsp. black pepper
- 1 tsp. garlic salt
- 2 tsp. Worcestershire sauce
- 8 oz. tomato sauce
- 2 garlic cloves, minced
- 1 small onion, chopped

Directions:
1. Grease a frying pan with cooking spray and fry the onion and garlic over a medium heat.
2. Stir in the beef, basil, chili powder, black pepper, and garlic salt, combining everything well. Allow to cook until the beef is nicely browned, before taking the pan off the heat.

3. Add in half of the cheese, the rice, Worcestershire sauce, and tomato sauce and stir to combine.
4. Spoon equal amounts of the beef mixture into the four bell peppers, filling them entirely.
5. Pre-heat the Air Fryer at 400°F.
6. Spritz the Air Fryer basket with cooking spray.
7. Put the stuffed bell peppers in the basket and allow to cook for 11 minutes.
8. Add the remaining cheese on top of each bell pepper with remaining cheese and cook for a further 2 minutes. When the cheese is melted and the bell peppers are piping hot, serve immediately.

315.Pesto Coated Rack Of Lamb

Servings:4
Cooking Time:15 Minutes
Ingredients:
- ½ bunch fresh mint
- 1 (1½-pounds) rack of lamb
- 1 garlic clove
- ¼ cup extra-virgin olive oil
- ½ tablespoon honey
- Salt and black pepper, to taste

Directions:
1. Preheat the Air fryer to 200 °F and grease an Air fryer basket.
2. Put the mint, garlic, oil, honey, salt, and black pepper in a blender and pulse until smooth to make pesto.
3. Coat the rack of lamb with this pesto on both sides and arrange in the Air fryer basket.
4. Cook for about 15 minutes and cut the rack into individual chops to serve.

316.Grilled Prosciutto Wrapped Fig

Servings:2
Cooking Time: 8 Minutes
Ingredients:
- 2 whole figs, sliced in quarters
- 8 prosciutto slices
- Pepper and salt to taste

Directions:
1. Wrap a prosciutto slice around one slice of fid and then thread into skewer. Repeat process for remaining Ingredients. Place on skewer rack in air fryer.
2. For 8 minutes, cook on 390 °F. Halfway through cooking time, turnover skewers.
3. Serve and enjoy.

317.Beef And Garlic Onions Sauce

Servings: 6
Cooking Time: 20 Minutes
Ingredients:
- 2-pound beef shank
- 1 teaspoon ground black pepper
- 1 teaspoon salt
- 1 oz crushed tomatoes
- 1 teaspoon sesame oil
- 3 tablespoons apple cider vinegar
- 1 garlic clove, diced
- 3 tablespoons water
- 3 spring onions, chopped

Directions:
1. Sprinkle the beef shank with ground black pepper and salt and put in the air fryer. Sprinkle the meat with sesame oil. Cook it for 20 minutes at 390F. Flip the meat on another side after 10 minutes of cooking. Meanwhile, make the sauce: put crushed tomatoes in the saucepan. Add apple cider vinegar, garlic clove, water, and spring onions. Bring the liquid to boil and remove it from the heat. When the meat is cooked, chop it into the servings and sprinkle with hot sauce.

318.Cheesy Herbs Burger Patties

Servings:2
Cooking Time: 25 Minutes
Ingredients:
- ¼ cup cheddar cheese
- ½ teaspoon dried rosemary, crushed
- 1-pound lean ground beef
- 2 green onions, sliced thinly
- 2 tablespoons chopped parsley
- 2 tablespoons ketchup
- 3 tablespoons Dijon mustard
- 3 tablespoons dry breadcrumbs
- Salt and pepper to taste

Directions:
1. In a mixing bowl, combine all ingredients except for the cheddar cheese.
2. Mix using your hands. Use your hands to make burger patties.
3. At the center of each patty, place a tablespoon of cheese and cover with the meat mixture.
4. Preheat the air fryer to 390°F.
5. Place the grill pan accessory and cook the patties for 25 minutes. Flip the patties halfway through the cooking time.

319.Spicy Mexican Beef With Cotija Cheese

Servings: 6
Cooking Time: 20 Minutes
Ingredients:
- 3 eggs, whisked
- 1/3 cup finely grated cotija cheese
- 1 cup parmesan cheese
- 6 minute steaks
- 2 tablespoons Mexican spice blend
- 1 ½ tablespoons olive oil

- Fine sea salt and ground black pepper, to taste

Directions:
1. Begin by sprinkling minute steaks with Mexican spice blend, salt and pepper.
2. Take a mixing dish and thoroughly combine the oil, cotija cheese, and parmesan cheese. In a separate mixing dish, beat the eggs.
3. Firstly, dip minute steaks in the egg; then, dip them in the cheese mixture.
4. Air-fry for 15 minutes at 345 degrees F; work in batches. Bon appétit!

320.Perfect Thai Meatballs

Servings:4
Cooking Time:20 Minutes
Ingredients:
- 1 pound ground beef
- 1 teaspoon red Thai curry paste
- 1/2 lime, rind and juice
- 1 teaspoon Chinese spice
- 2 teaspoons lemongrass, finely chopped
- 1 tablespoon sesame oil

Directions:
1. Thoroughly combine all ingredients in a mixing dish.
2. Shape into 24 meatballs and place them into the Air Fryer cooking basket. Cook at 380 degrees F for 10 minutes; pause the machine and cook for a further 5 minutes, or until cooked through.
3. Serve accompanied by the dipping sauce. Bon appétit!

321.Tasty Beef Pot Pie

Servings:6
Cooking Time: 30 Minutes
Ingredients:
- 1 cup almond flour
- 1 green bell pepper, julienned
- 1 onion, chopped
- 1 red bell pepper, julienned
- 1 tablespoon butter
- 1 yellow bell pepper, julienned
- 1-pound ground beef
- 2 beaten eggs
- 2 cloves of garlic, minced
- 4 tablespoons coconut oil
- Salt and pepper to taste

Directions:
1. Preheat the air fryer for 5 minutes.
2. In a baking dish that will fit in the air fryer, combine the first 9 ingredients. Mix well then set aside.
3. In a mixing bowl, mix the almond flour and eggs to create a dough.
4. Press the dough over the beef mixture.
5. Place in the air fryer and cook for 30 minutes at 350°F.

322.Nana's Pork Chops With Cilantro

Servings: 6
Cooking Time: 22 Minutes
Ingredients:
- 1/3 cup pork rinds
- Roughly chopped fresh cilantro, to taste
- 2 teaspoons Cajun seasonings
- Nonstick cooking spray
- 2 eggs, beaten
- 3 tablespoons almond meal
- 1 teaspoon seasoned salt
- Garlic & onion spice blend, to taste
- 6 pork chops
- 1/3 teaspoon freshly cracked black pepper

Directions:
1. Coat the pork chops with Cajun seasonings, salt, pepper, and the spice blend on all sides.
2. Then, add the almond meal to a plate. In a shallow dish, whisk the egg until pale and smooth. Place the pork rinds in the third bowl.
3. Dredge each pork piece in the almond meal; then, coat them with the egg; finally, coat them with the pork rinds. Spritz them with cooking spray on both sides.
4. Now, air-fry pork chops for about 18 minutes at 345 degrees F; make sure to taste for doneness after first 12 minutes of cooking. Lastly, garnish with fresh cilantro. Bon appétit!

323.Glazed Ham

Servings:4
Cooking Time:40 Minutes
Ingredients:
- 1 pound (10½ ounce) ham joint
- ¾ cup whiskey
- 2 tablespoons French mustard
- 2 tablespoons honey

Directions:
1. Preheat the Air fryer to 320 °F and grease an Air fryer pan.
2. Mix all the ingredients in a bowl except ham.
3. Keep ham joint for about 30 minutes at room temperature and place in the Air fryer pan.
4. Top with half of the whiskey mixture and transfer into the Air fryer.
5. Cook for about 15 minutes and flip the side.
6. Coat with the remaining whiskey mixture and cook for about 25 minutes.
7. Dish out in a platter and serve warm.

324.Honey Mustard Cheesy Meatballs

Servings:8
Cooking Time:15 Minutes
Ingredients:
- 2 onions, chopped
- 1 pound ground beef

- 4 tablespoons fresh basil, chopped
- 2 tablespoons cheddar cheese, grated
- 2 teaspoons garlic paste
- 2 teaspoons honey
- Salt and black pepper, to taste
- 2 teaspoons mustard

Directions:
1. Preheat the Air fryer to 385 °F and grease an Air fryer basket.
2. Mix all the ingredients in a bowl until well combined.
3. Shape the mixture into equal-sized balls gently and arrange the meatballs in the Air fryer basket.
4. Cook for about 15 minutes and dish out to serve warm.

325.Another Easy Teriyaki Bbq Recipe

Servings:2
Cooking Time: 15 Minutes
Ingredients:
- 1 tbsp honey
- 1 tbsp mirin
- 1 tbsp soy sauce
- 1 thumb-sized piece of fresh ginger, grated
- 14 oz lean diced steak, with fat trimmed

Directions:
1. Mix all Ingredients in a bowl and marinate for at least an hour. Turning over halfway through marinating time.
2. Thread mead into skewers. Place on skewer rack.
3. Cook for 5 minutes at 390 °F or to desired doneness.
4. Serve and enjoy.

326.Smoked Pork

Servings: 5
Cooking Time: 20 Minutes
Ingredients:
- 1-pound pork shoulder
- 1 tablespoon liquid smoke
- 1 tablespoon olive oil
- 1 teaspoon salt

Directions:
1. Mix up liquid smoke, salt, and olive oil in the shallow bowl. Then carefully brush the pork shoulder with the liquid smoke mixture from each side. Make the small cuts in the meat. Preheat the air fryer to 390F. Put the pork shoulder in the air fryer basket and cook the meat for 10 minutes. After this, flip the meat on another side and cook it for 10 minutes more. Let the cooked pork shoulder rest for 10-15 minutes. Shred it with the help of 2 forks.

327.Hickory Smoked Beef Jerky

Servings:2

Cooking Time: 1 Hour
Ingredients:
- ¼ cup Worcestershire sauce
- ½ cup brown sugar
- ½ cup soy sauce
- ½ teaspoon black pepper
- ½ teaspoon smoked paprika
- 1 tablespoon chili pepper sauce
- 1 tablespoon liquid smoke, hickory
- 1 teaspoon garlic powder
- 1 teaspoon onion powder
- 1-pound ground beef, sliced thinly

Directions:
1. Combine all Ingredients in a mixing bowl or Ziploc bag.
2. Marinate in the fridge overnight.
3. Preheat the air fryer to 330°F.
4. Place the beef slices on the double layer rack.
5. Cook for one hour until the beef jerky is very dry.

328.Dill Pork Shoulder

Servings: 4
Cooking Time: 20 Minutes
Ingredients:
- 1-pound pork shoulder, boneless
- 3 spring onions, chopped
- 1 teaspoon dried dill
- 1 teaspoon keto tomato sauce
- 1 tablespoon water
- 1 teaspoon salt
- 2 tablespoons sesame oil
- 1 teaspoon ground black pepper
- ½ teaspoon garlic powder

Directions:
1. In the shallow bowl mix up salt, ground black pepper, and garlic powder. Then add dried dill. Sprinkle the pork shoulder with a spice mixture from each side. Then in the separated bowl, mix up tomato sauce, water, and sesame oil. Brush the meat with the tomato mixture. Then place it on the foil. Add spring onions. Wrap the pork shoulder. Preheat the air fryer to 395F. Put the wrapped pork shoulder in the air fryer basket and cook it for 20 minutes. Let the cooked meat rest for 5-10 minutes and then discard the foil.

329.Pork Ribs With Red Wine Sauce

Servings: 4
Cooking Time: 25 Minutes + Marinating Time
Ingredients:
- For the Pork Ribs:
- 1 ½ pounds pork ribs
- 2 tablespoons olive oil
- 1/2 teaspoon freshly cracked black peppercorns

- 1/2 teaspoon Hickory-smoked salt
- 1 tablespoon Dijon mustard
- 2 tablespoons coconut aminos
- 2 tablespoons lime juice
- 1 clove garlic, minced
- For the Red Wine Sauce:
- 1 ½ cups beef stock
- 1 cup red wine
- 1 teaspoon balsamic vinegar
- 1/4 teaspoon salt

Directions:
1. Place all ingredients for the pork ribs in a large-sized mixing dish. Cover and marinate in your refrigerator overnight or at least 3 hours.
2. Air-fry the pork ribs for 10 minutes at 320 degrees F.
3. Meanwhile, make the sauce. Add a beef stock to a deep pan that is preheated over a moderate flame; boil until it is reduced by half.
4. Add the remaining ingredients and increase the temperature to high heat. Let it cook for further 10 minutes or until your sauce is reduced by half.
5. Serve the pork ribs with red wine sauce. Bon appétit!

330.Easy & The Traditional Beef Roast Recipe

Servings:12
Cooking Time: 2 Hours
Ingredients:
- 1 cup organic beef broth
- 3 pounds beef round roast
- 4 tablespoons olive oil
- Salt and pepper to taste

Directions:
1. Place in a Ziploc bag all the ingredients and allow to marinate in the fridge for 2 hours.
2. Preheat the air fryer for 5 minutes.
3. Transfer all ingredients in a baking dish that will fit in the air fryer.
4. Place in the air fryer and cook for 2 hours for 400°F.

331.Creamy Burger & Potato Bake

Servings:3
Cooking Time: 55 Minutes
Ingredients:
- salt to taste
- freshly ground pepper, to taste
- 1/2 (10.75 ounce) can condensed cream of mushroom soup
- 1/2-pound lean ground beef
- 1-1/2 cups peeled and thinly sliced potatoes
- 1/2 cup shredded Cheddar cheese
- 1/4 cup chopped onion

- 1/4 cup and 2 tablespoons milk

Directions:
1. Lightly grease baking pan of air fryer with cooking spray. Add ground beef. For 10 minutes, cook on 360 °F. Stir and crumble halfway through cooking time.
2. Meanwhile, in a bowl, whisk well pepper, salt, milk, onion, and mushroom soup. Mix well.
3. Drain fat off ground beef and transfer beef to a plate.
4. In same air fryer baking pan, layer ½ of potatoes on bottom, then ½ of soup mixture, and then ½ of beef. Repeat process.
5. Cover pan with foil.
6. Cook for 30 minutes. Remove foil and cook for another 15 minutes or until potatoes are tender.
7. Serve and enjoy.

332.Charred Onions 'n Steak Cube Bbq

Servings:3
Cooking Time: 40 Minutes
Ingredients:
- 1 cup red onions, cut into wedges
- 1 tablespoon dry mustard
- 1 tablespoon olive oil
- 1-pound boneless beef sirloin, cut into cubes
- Salt and pepper to taste

Directions:
1. Preheat the air fryer to 390°F.
2. Place the grill pan accessory in the air fryer.
3. Toss all ingredients in a bowl and mix until everything is coated with the seasonings.
4. Place on the grill pan and cook for 40 minutes.
5. Halfway through the cooking time, give a stir to cook evenly.

333.Coconut Pork And Green Beans

Servings: 4
Cooking Time: 25 Minutes
Ingredients:
- 4 pork chops
- 2 tablespoons coconut oil, melted
- 2 garlic cloves, minced
- A pinch of salt and black pepper
- ½ pound green beans, trimmed and halved
- 2 tablespoons keto tomato sauce

Directions:
1. Heat up a pan that fits the air fryer with the oil over medium heat, add the pork chops and brown for 5 minutes. Add the rest of the ingredients, put the pan in the machine and cook at 390 degrees F for 20 minutes. Divide everything between plates and serve

334.Spiced Lamb Steaks

Servings:3
Cooking Time:15 Minutes
Ingredients:
- ½ onion, roughly chopped
- 1½ pounds boneless lamb sirloin steaks
- 5 garlic cloves, peeled
- 1 tablespoon fresh ginger, peeled
- 1 teaspoon garam masala
- 1 teaspoon ground fennel
- ½ teaspoon ground cumin
- ½ teaspoon ground cinnamon
- ½ teaspoon cayenne pepper
- Salt and black pepper, to taste

Directions:
1. Preheat the Air fryer to 330 °F and grease an Air fryer basket.
2. Put the onion, garlic, ginger, and spices in a blender and pulse until smooth.
3. Coat the lamb steaks with this mixture on both sides and refrigerate to marinate for about 24 hours.
4. Arrange the lamb steaks in the Air fryer basket and cook for about 15 minutes, flipping once in between.
5. Dish out the steaks in a platter and serve warm.

335.Italian Twisted Pork Chops

Servings: 3
Cooking Time: 20 Minutes
Ingredients:
- 1/4 cup balsamic vinegar
- 3 center-cut loin pork chops
- 1/4 cup almond meal
- 2 tablespoons golden flaxseed meal
- 1 teaspoon turmeric powder
- 1 egg
- 1 teaspoon mustard
- Kosher salt, to taste
- 1/4 teaspoon freshly ground black pepper
- 1/2 cup pork rinds, crushed
- 1/2 teaspoon garlic powder
- 1 teaspoon shallot powder

Directions:
1. Drizzle the balsamic vinegar over pork chops and spread to evenly coat.
2. Place the almond meal, flaxseed meal, and turmeric in a shallow bowl. In another bowl, whisk the eggs, mustard, salt, and black pepper.
3. In the third bowl, mix the pork rinds with the garlic powder and shallot powder.
4. Preheat your Air Fryer to 390 degrees F. Dredge the pork chops in the almond meal mixture, then in the egg, followed by the pork rind mixture.
5. Cook the pork chops for 7 minutes per side, spraying with cooking oil. Bon appétit!

336.Beef & Kale Omelet

Servings: 4
Cooking Time: 20 Minutes
Ingredients:
- Cooking spray
- ½ lb. leftover beef, coarsely chopped
- 2 garlic cloves, pressed
- 1 cup kale, torn into pieces and wilted
- 1 tomato, chopped
- ¼ tsp. sugar
- 4 eggs, beaten
- 4 tbsp. heavy cream
- ½ tsp. turmeric powder
- Salt and ground black pepper to taste
- 1/8 tsp. ground allspice

Directions:
1. Grease four ramekins with cooking spray.
2. Place equal amounts of each of the ingredients into each ramekin and mix well.
3. Air-fry at 360°F for 16 minutes, or longer if necessary. Serve immediately.

337.Spicy Lamb Kebabs

Servings:6
Cooking Time:8 Minutes
Ingredients:
- 4 eggs, beaten
- 1 cup pistachios, chopped
- 1 pound ground lamb
- 4 tablespoons plain flour
- 4 tablespoons flat-leaf parsley, chopped
- 2 teaspoons chili flakes
- 4 garlic cloves, minced
- 2 tablespoons fresh lemon juice
- 2 teaspoons cumin seeds
- 1 teaspoon fennel seeds
- 2 teaspoons dried mint
- 2 teaspoons salt
- Olive oil
- 1 teaspoon coriander seeds
- 1 teaspoon freshly ground black pepper

Directions:
1. Preheat the Air fryer to 355 °F and grease an Air fryer basket.
2. Mix lamb, pistachios, eggs, lemon juice, chili flakes, flour, cumin seeds, fennel seeds, coriander seeds, mint, parsley, salt and black pepper in a large bowl.
3. Thread the lamb mixture onto metal skewers to form sausages and coat with olive oil.
4. Place the skewers in the Air fryer basket and cook for about 8 minutes.
5. Dish out in a platter and serve hot.

338.Flavorsome Pork Chops With Peanut Sauce

Servings:4

Cooking Time:12 Minutes
Ingredients:
- 1 pound pork chops, cubed into 1-inch size
- 1 shallot, chopped finely
- ¾ cup ground peanuts
- ¾ cup coconut milk
- For Pork:
- 1 teaspoon fresh ginger, minced
- 1 garlic clove, minced
- 2 tablespoon soy sauce
- 1 tablespoon olive oil
- 1 teaspoon hot pepper sauce
- For Peanut Sauce:
- 1 tablespoon olive oil
- 1 garlic clove, minced
- 1 teaspoon ground coriander
- 1 tablespoon olive oil
- 1 teaspoon hot pepper sauce

Directions:
1. Preheat the Air fryer to 390 °F and grease an Air fryer basket.
2. For Pork:
3. Mix all the ingredients in a bowl and keep aside for about 30 minutes.
4. Arrange the chops in the Air fryer basket and cook for about 12 minutes, flipping once in between.
5. For Peanut Sauce:
6. Heat olive oil in a pan on medium heat and add shallot and garlic.
7. Sauté for about 3 minutes and stir in coriander.
8. Sauté for about 1 minute and add rest of the ingredients.
9. Cook for about 5 minutes and pour over the pork chops to serve.

339.American Garlic Ribs

Servings: 4
Cooking Time: 30 Minutes
Ingredients:
- 11-pound pork spare ribs
- ¼ cup keto tomato sauce
- 1 tablespoon lemon juice
- 1 tablespoon avocado oil
- 1 teaspoon Splenda
- 1 tablespoon American style yellow mustard
- ½ teaspoon minced garlic
- 1 teaspoon chili pepper
- ½ teaspoon ground black pepper

Directions:
1. In the mixing bowl mix up tomato sauce, lemon juice, avocado oil, Splenda, yellow mustard, minced garlic, chili pepper, and ground black pepper. Stir the mixture until homogenous. Then rub the spare ribs with the mustard mixture and leave for 20 minutes to marinate. Preheat the air fryer to 355F and place the marinated spare ribs in the air fryer basket. Cook the meal for 30 minutes.

340.Italian Fennel Lamb

Servings: 6
Cooking Time: 22 Minutes
Ingredients:
- 18 oz rack of lamb
- 1 teaspoon Italian seasonings
- ½ teaspoon cayenne pepper
- ½ teaspoon dried thyme
- ½ teaspoon dried cumin
- 1 teaspoon fennel seeds
- ½ teaspoon lemon zest, grated
- 1 tablespoon coconut oil, melted
- ½ teaspoon onion powder

Directions:
1. Sprinkle the rack of lamb with Italian seasonings, cayenne pepper, dried thyme, cumin, fennel seeds, and onion powder. Then sprinkle the meat with lemon zest and coconut oil. Preheat the air fryer to 385F. Put the rack off the lamb in the air fryer basket and cook it for 22 minutes.

341.Beef Cheeseburgers

Servings:2
Cooking Time:12 Minutes
Ingredients:
- ½ pound ground beef
- 2 tablespoons fresh cilantro, minced
- 2 slices cheddar cheese
- 2 salad leaves
- 2 dinner rolls, cut into half
- 1 garlic clove, minced
- Salt and black pepper, to taste

Directions:
1. Preheat the Air fryer to 390 °F and grease an Air fryer basket.
2. Mix the beef, garlic, cilantro, salt, and black pepper in a bowl.
3. Make 2 equal-sized patties from the beef mixture and arrange in the Air fryer basket.
4. Cook for about 11 minutes and top each patty with 1 cheese slice.
5. Cook for about 1 more minute and dish out in a platter.
6. Place dinner rolls in a serving platter and arrange salad leaf between each dinner roll.
7. Top with 1 patty and immediately serve

342.Herb-crusted Filet Mignon

Servings: 4
Cooking Time: 20 Minutes
Ingredients:
- 1 pound filet mignon
- Sea salt and ground black pepper, to your liking

- 1/2 teaspoon cayenne pepper
- 1 teaspoon dried basil
- 1 teaspoon dried rosemary
- 1 teaspoon dried thyme
- 1 tablespoon sesame oil
- 1 small-sized egg, well-whisked
- 1/2 cup parmesan cheese, grated

Directions:
1. Season the filet mignon with salt, black pepper, cayenne pepper, basil, rosemary, and thyme. Brush with sesame oil.
2. Put the egg in a shallow plate. Now, place the parmesan cheese in another plate.
3. Coat the filet mignon with the egg; then, lay it into the parmesan cheese. Set your Air Fryer to cook at 360 degrees F.
4. Cook for 10 to 13 minutes or until golden. Serve with mixed salad leaves and enjoy!

343.Garlic Pork Medallions

Servings: 4
Cooking Time: 50 Minutes
Ingredients:
- 1-pound pork loin
- 2 tablespoons apple cider vinegar
- 2 tablespoons lemon juice
- ¼ cup heavy cream
- 1 teaspoon salt
- 1 teaspoon white pepper
- 1 garlic clove, diced
- 3 spring onions, diced
- 1 teaspoon lemon zest, grated
- 2 tablespoons avocado oil

Directions:
1. Make the marinade: in the mixing bowl mix up apple cider vinegar, lemon juice, heavy cream, salt, white pepper, diced garlic, onion, and lemon zest. Then add avocado oil and whisk the marinade carefully. Chop the pork loin roughly and put in the marinade. Coat the meat in the marinade carefully (use the spoon for this) and leave it for 20 minutes in the fridge. Meanwhile, preheat the air fryer to 365F. Put the marinated meat in the air fryer and cook it for 50 minutes. Stir the meat during cooking to avoid burning.

344.Pork Chops Marinate In Honey-mustard

Servings:4
Cooking Time: 25 Minutes
Ingredients:
- 2 tablespoons honey
- 2 tablespoons minced garlic
- 4 pork chops
- 4 tablespoons mustard
- Salt and pepper to taste

Directions:
1. Preheat the air fryer to 330°F.
2. Place the air fryer basket.

3. Season the pork chops with the rest of the Ingredients.
4. Place inside the basket.
5. Cook for 20 to 25 minutes until golden.

345.Garlic Lamb Roast

Servings:6
Cooking Time: 1½ Hours
Ingredients:
- 2¾ pounds half lamb leg roast
- 3 garlic cloves, cut into thin slices
- 2 tablespoons extra-virgin olive oil
- 1 tablespoon dried rosemary, crushed
- Salt and ground black pepper, as required

Directions:
1. In a small bowl, mix together the oil, rosemary, salt, and black pepper.
2. With the tip of a sharp knife, make deep slits on the top of lamb roast fat.
3. Insert the garlic slices into the slits.
4. Coat the lamb roast evenly with oil mixture.
5. Set the temperature of air fryer to 390 degrees F. Grease an air fryer basket.
6. Arrange lamb into the prepared air fryer basket in a single layer.
7. Air Fry for about 15 minutes and then another 1¼ hours at 320 degrees F.
8. Remove from air fryer and transfer the roast onto a platter.
9. With a piece of foil, cover the roast for about 10 minutes before slicing.
10. Cut the roast into desired size slices and serve.

346.Pork And Peppers Mix

Servings: 4
Cooking Time: 25 Minutes
Ingredients:
- 1 pound pork tenderloin, sliced
- ¼ cup cilantro, chopped
- ½ teaspoon garlic powder
- 1 tablespoon olive oil
- 1 green bell pepper, julienned
- ½ teaspoon chili powder
- ½ teaspoon cumin, ground

Directions:
1. Heat up a pan that fits the air fryer with the oil over medium heat, add the pork and brown for 5 minutes. Add the rest of the ingredients, toss, put the pan in the air fryer and cook at 400 degrees F for 20 minutes. Divide between plates and serve.

347.Fried Sausage And Mushrooms Recipe

Servings: 6
Cooking Time:50 Minutes
Ingredients:
- 3 red bell peppers; chopped
- 2 sweet onions; chopped.
- 1 tbsp. brown sugar
- 1 tsp. olive oil
- 2 lbs. pork sausage; sliced

- Salt and black pepper to the taste
- 2 lbs. Portobello mushrooms; sliced

Directions:
1. In a baking dish that fits your air fryer, mix sausage slices with oil, salt, pepper, bell pepper, mushrooms, onion and sugar, toss, introduce in your air fryer and cook at 300 °F, for 40 minutes. Divide among plates and serve right away.

348.Salted 'n Peppered Scored Beef Chuck

Servings:6
Cooking Time: 1 Hour And 30 Minutes
Ingredients:
- 2 ounces black peppercorns
- 2 tablespoons olive oil
- 3 pounds beef chuck roll, scored with knife
- 3 tablespoons salt

Directions:
1. Preheat the air fryer to 390°F.
2. Place the grill pan accessory in the air fryer.
3. Season the beef chuck roll with black peppercorns and salt.
4. Brush with olive oil and cover top with foil.
5. Grill for 1 hour and 30 minutes.
6. Flip the beef every 30 minutes for even grilling on all sides.

349.Simple Herbs De Provence Pork Loin Roast

Servings:4
Cooking Time: 35 Minutes
Ingredients:
- 4 pounds pork loin
- A pinch of garlic salt
- A pinch of herbs de Provence

Directions:
1. Preheat the air fryer to 330°F.
2. Season pork with the garlic salt and herbs,
3. Place in the air fryer grill pan.
4. Cook for 30 to 35 minutes.

350.Beef With Tomato Sauce And Fennel

Servings: 4
Cooking Time: 20 Minutes
Ingredients:
- 2 tablespoons olive oil
- 1 pound beef, cut into strips
- 1 fennel bulb, sliced
- Salt and black pepper to the taste
- 1 teaspoon sweet paprika
- ¼ cup keto tomato sauce

Directions:
1. Heat up a pan that fits the air fryer with the oil over medium-high heat, add the beef and brown for 5 minutes. Add the rest of the ingredients, toss, put the pan in the machine and cook at 380 degrees F for 15 minutes. Divide the mix between plates and serve.

351.Classic Smoked Pork Chops

Servings: 6

Cooking Time: 25 Minutes
Ingredients:
- 6 pork chops
- Hickory-smoked salt, to savor
- Ground black pepper, to savor
- 1 teaspoon onion powder
- 1/2 teaspoon garlic powder
- 1/2 teaspoon cayenne pepper
- 1/3 cup almond meal

Directions:
1. Simply place all of the above ingredients into a zip-top plastic bag; shake them up to coat well.
2. Spritz the chops with a pan spray (canola spray works well here) and transfer them to the Air Fryer cooking basket.
3. Roast them for 20 minutes at 375 degrees F. Serve with sautéed vegetables. Bon appétit!

352.Lamb Chops With Veggies

Servings:4
Cooking Time: 8 Minutes
Ingredients:
- 2 tablespoons fresh rosemary, minced
- 2 tablespoons fresh mint leaves, minced
- 1 garlic clove, minced
- 3 tablespoons olive oil
- Salt and ground black pepper, as required
- 4 (6-ounces) lamb chops
- 1 purple carrot, peeled and cubed
- 1 yellow carrot, peeled and cubed
- 1 parsnip, peeled and cubed
- 1 fennel bulb, cubed

Directions:
1. In a large bowl, mix together the herbs, garlic, oil, salt, and black pepper.
2. Add the chops and generously coat with mixture.
3. Refrigerate to marinate for about 3 hours.
4. In a large pan of water, soak the vegetables for about 15 minutes.
5. Drain the vegetables completely.
6. Set the temperature of air fryer to 390 degrees F. Grease an air fryer basket.
7. Arrange chops into the prepared air fryer basket in a single layer.
8. Air Fry for about 2 minutes.
9. Remove chops from the air fryer.
10. Place vegetables into the air fryer basket and top with the chops in a single layer.
11. Air Fry for about 6 minutes.
12. Remove from air fryer and transfer the chops and vegetables onto serving plates.
13. Serve hot.

353.Festive Teriyaki Beef

Servings:4
Cooking Time:40 Minutes
Ingredients:
- 2 heaping tablespoons fresh parsley, roughly chopped
- 1 pound beef rump steaks

- 2 heaping tablespoons fresh chives, roughly chopped
- Salt and black pepper (or mixed peppercorns, to savor
- For the Sauce:
- ½ cup grapefruit juice
- 1/3 cup hoisin sauce
- 1 tablespoon fresh ginger, grated
- 1 ½ tablespoons mirin
- 3 garlic cloves, minced
- 2 tablespoon rice bran oil
- ½ cup soy sauce
- 1/3 cup brown sugar

Directions:
1. Firstly, steam the beef rump steaks for 8 minutes (use the method of steaming that you prefer. Season the beef with salt and black pepper; scatter the chopped parsley and chives over the top.
2. Roast the beef rump steaks in an air fryer basket for 28 minutes at 345 degrees, turning halfway through.
3. While the beef is cooking, combine the ingredients for the teriyaki sauce in a sauté pan. Then, let it simmer over low heat until it has thickened.
4. Toss the beef with the teriyaki sauce until it is well covered and serve.

354.Herbs Crumbed Rack Of Lamb

Servings:5
Cooking Time: 30 Minutes
Ingredients:
- 1 tablespoon butter, melted
- 1 garlic clove, finely chopped
- 1¾ pounds rack of lamb
- Salt and ground black pepper, as required
- 1 egg
- ½ cup panko breadcrumbs
- 1 tablespoon fresh thyme, minced
- 1 tablespoon fresh rosemary, minced

Directions:
1. In a bowl, mix together the butter, garlic, salt, and black pepper.
2. Coat the rack of lamb evenly with garlic mixture.
3. In a shallow dish, beat the egg.
4. In another dish, mix together the breadcrumbs and herbs.
5. Dip the rack of lamb in beaten egg and then, coat with breadcrumbs mixture.
6. Set the temperature of air fryer to 212 degrees F. Grease an air fryer basket.
7. Place rack of lamb into the prepared air fryer basket.
8. Air Fry for about 25 minutes and then 5 more minutes at 390 degrees F.
9. Remove from air fryer and place the rack of lamb onto a cutting board for about 5 minutes
10. With a sharp knife, cut the rack of lamb into individual chops and serve.

355.Easy Rib Eye Steak

Servings:4
Cooking Time:14 Minutes
Ingredients:
- 2 lbs. rib eye steak
- 1 tablespoon olive oil
- 1 tablespoon steak rubo

Directions:
1. Preheat the Air fryer to 400 °F and grease an Air fryer basket.
2. Rub the steak generously with steak rub and coat with olive oil.
3. Transfer the steak in the Air fryer basket and cook for about 14 minutes, flipping once in between.
4. Dish out the steak and cut into desired size slices to serve.

356.German Schnitzel

Servings: 4
Cooking Time: 15 Minutes
Ingredients:
- 4 thin beef schnitzel
- 1 tbsp. sesame seeds
- 2 tbsp. paprika
- 3 tbsp. olive oil
- 4 tbsp. flour
- 2 eggs, beaten
- 1 cup friendly bread crumbs
- Pepper and salt to taste

Directions:
1. Pre-heat the Air Fryer at 350°F.
2. Sprinkle the pepper and salt on the schnitzel.
3. In a shallow dish, combine the paprika, flour, and salt
4. In a second shallow dish, mix the bread crumbs with the sesame seeds.
5. Place the beaten eggs in a bowl.
6. Coat the schnitzel in the flour mixture. Dip it into the egg before rolling it in the bread crumbs.
7. Put the coated schnitzel in the Air Fryer basket and allow to cook for 12 minutes before serving hot.

357.Air Fried Grilled Steak

Servings:2
Cooking Time: 45 Minutes
Ingredients:
- 2 top sirloin steaks
- 3 tablespoons butter, melted
- 3 tablespoons olive oil
- Salt and pepper to taste

Directions:
1. Preheat the air fryer for 5 minutes.
2. Season the sirloin steaks with olive oil, salt and pepper.
3. Place the beef in the air fryer basket.
4. Cook for 45 minutes at 350°F.
5. Once cooked, serve with butter.

358.Cumin-sichuan Lamb Bbq With Dip

Servings:4
Cooking Time: 25 Minutes
Directions:
1. In a food processor, process cumin seeds, peppercorns, caraway seeds, pepper flakes, and sugar until smooth.
2. Thread lamb pieces into skewers. Season with salt. Rub paste all over meat pieces.
3. Place on skewer rack.
4. Cook for 5 minutes at 390 °F or to desired doneness.
5. Meanwhile, in a medium bowl whisk well dip Ingredients and set aside.
6. Serve and enjoy with dip.

359.Traditional Beef 'n Tomato Stew

Servings:4
Cooking Time: 40 Minutes
Ingredients:
- 2 tablespoons quick-cooking tapioca
- 1 teaspoon sugar
- 1 teaspoons salt
- 1-pound beef stew meat, cut into 1-inch cubes
- 2 medium carrots, cut into 1-inch chunks
- 1 large potato, peeled and quartered
- 1 small onion, cut into chunks
- 1 slice bread, cubed
- 1/2 can (14-1/2 ounces) diced tomatoes, undrained
- 1/2 cup water
- 1/2 teaspoon pepper
- 1 celery rib, cut into 3/4-inch chunks

Directions:
1. Lightly grease baking pan of air fryer with cooking spray. Add all Ingredients and toss well to coat.
2. Cover pan with foil.
3. For 25 minutes, cook on 390 °F. Halfway through cooking time, stir.
4. Remove foil, stir well, and cook for 15 minutes at 330 °F.
5. Serve and enjoy.

360.Air Fryer Beef Casserole

Servings:4
Cooking Time: 30 Minutes
Ingredients:
- 1 green bell pepper, seeded and chopped
- 1 onion, chopped
- 1-pound ground beef
- 3 cloves of garlic, minced
- 3 tablespoons olive oil
- 6 cups eggs, beaten
- Salt and pepper to taste

Directions:
1. Preheat the air fryer for 5 minutes.
2. In a baking dish that will fit in the air fryer, mix the ground beef, onion, garlic, olive oil, and bell pepper. Season with salt and pepper to taste.
3. Pour in the beaten eggs and give a good stir.
4. Place the dish with the beef and egg mixture in the air fryer.
5. Bake for 30 minutes at 325°F.

361.Herbed Pork Burgers

Servings:8
Cooking Time:45 Minutes
Ingredients:
- 2 small onions, chopped
- 21-ounce ground pork
- 2 teaspoons fresh basil, chopped
- 8 burger buns
- ½ cup cheddar cheese, grated
- 2 teaspoons mustard
- 2 teaspoons garlic puree
- 2 teaspoons tomato puree
- Salt and freshly ground black pepper, to taste
- 2 teaspoons dried mixed herbs, crushed

Directions:
1. Preheat the Air fryer to 395 °F and grease an Air fryer basket.
2. Mix all the ingredients in a bowl except cheese and buns.
3. Make 8 equal-sized patties from the pork mixture and arrange thee patties in the Air fryer basket.
4. Cook for about 45 minutes, flipping once in between and arrange the patties in buns with cheese to serve.

362.Italian Beef Meatballs

Servings:6
Cooking Time:15 Minutes
Ingredients:
- 2 large eggs
- 2 pounds ground beef
- ¼ cup fresh parsley, chopped
- 1¼ cups panko breadcrumbs
- ¼ cup Parmigiano Reggiano, grated
- 1 teaspoon dried oregano
- 1 small garlic clove, chopped
- Salt and black pepper, to taste
- 1 teaspoon vegetable oil

Directions:
1. Preheat the Air fryer to 350 °F and grease an Air fryer basket.
2. Mix beef with all other ingredients in a bowl until well combined.
3. Make equal-sized balls from the mixture and arrange the balls in the Air fryer basket.
4. Cook for about 13 minutes and dish out to serve warm.

363.Lamb Burgers

Servings: 2
Cooking Time: 16 Minutes
Ingredients:
- 8 oz lamb, minced
- ½ teaspoon salt
- ½ teaspoon ground black pepper

- ½ teaspoon dried cilantro
- 1 tablespoon water
- Cooking spray

Directions:
1. In the mixing bowl mix up minced lamb, salt, ground black pepper, dried cilantro, and water.
2. Stir the meat mixture carefully with the help of the spoon and make 2 burgers.
3. Preheat the air fryer to 375F.
4. Spray the air fryer basket with cooking spray and put the burgers inside.
5. Cook them for 8 minutes from each side.

364.Pork Chops With Peanut Sauce

Servings:4
Cooking Time: 12 Minutes
Ingredients:
- For Chops:
- 1 teaspoon fresh ginger, minced
- 1 garlic clove, minced
- 2 tablespoons soy sauce
- 1 tablespoon olive oil
- 1 teaspoon hot pepper sauce
- 1-pound boneless pork chop, cubed into 1-inch size
- For Peanut Sauce:
- 1 tablespoon olive oil
- 1 shallot, finely chopped
- 1 garlic clove, minced
- 1 teaspoon ground coriander
- ¾ cup ground peanuts
- 1 teaspoon hot pepper sauce
- ¾ cup coconut milk

Directions:
1. For pork: in a bowl, mix together the ginger, garlic, soy sauce, oil, and hot pepper sauce.
2. Add the pork chops and generously coat with mixture.
3. Place at the room temperature for about 15 minutes.
4. Set the temperature of air fryer to 390 degrees F. Grease an air fryer basket.
5. Arrange chops into the prepared air fryer basket in a single layer.
6. Air fry for about 12 minutes.
7. Meanwhile, for the sauce: in a pan, heat oil over medium heat and sauté the shallot and garlic for about 2-3 minutes.
8. Add the coriander and sauté for about 1 minute.
9. Stir in the remaining ingredients and cook for about 5 minutes, stirring continuously.
10. Remove the pan of sauce from heat and let it cool slightly.
11. Remove the chops from air fryer and transfer onto serving plates.
12. Serve immediately with the topping of peanut sauce.

365.Grilled Steak On Tomato-olive Salad

Servings:5
Cooking Time: 50 Minutes
Ingredients:
- ¼ cup extra virgin olive oil
- ¼ teaspoon cayenne pepper
- ½ cup green olives, pitted and sliced
- 1 cup red onion, chopped
- 1 tablespoon oil
- 1 teaspoon paprika
- 2 ½ pound flank
- 2 pounds cherry tomatoes, halved
- 2 tablespoons Sherry vinegar
- Salt and pepper to taste

Directions:
1. Preheat the air fryer to 390°F.
2. Place the grill pan accessory in the air fryer.
3. Season the steak with salt, pepper, paprika, and cayenne pepper. Brush with oil
4. Place on the grill pan and cook for 45 to 50 minutes.
5. Meanwhile, prepare the salad by mixing the remaining ingredients.
6. Serve the beef with salad.

366.Salt And Pepper Pork Chinese Style

Servings:4
Cooking Time: 25 Minutes
Ingredients:
- ½ teaspoon sea salt
- ¾ cup potato starch
- 1 egg white, beaten
- 1 red bell pepper, chopped
- 1 teaspoon Chinese five-spice powder
- 1 teaspoon sesame oil
- 2 green bell peppers, chopped
- 2 tablespoons toasted sesame seeds
- 4 pork chops

Directions:
1. Preheat the air fryer to 330°F.
2. Season the pork chops with salt and five spice powder.
3. Dip in egg white and dredge in potato starch.
4. Place in the air fryer basket and cook for 25 minutes.
5. Meanwhile, heat oil in a skillet and stir-fry the bell peppers.
6. Serve the bell peppers on top of pork chops and garnish with sesame seeds.

FISH & SEAFOOD RECIPES

367.Catfish With Spring Onions And Avocado

Servings: 4
Cooking Time: 15 Minutes
Ingredients:
- 2 teaspoons oregano, dried
- 2 teaspoons cumin, ground
- 2 teaspoons sweet paprika
- A pinch of salt and black pepper
- 4 catfish fillets
- 1 avocado, peeled and cubed
- ½ cup spring onions, chopped
- 2 tablespoons cilantro, chopped
- 2 teaspoons olive oil
- 2 tablespoons lemon juice

Directions:
1. In a bowl, mix all the ingredients except the fish and toss. Arrange this in a baking pan that fits the air fryer, top with the fish, introduce the pan in the machine and cook at 360 degrees F for 15 minutes, flipping the fish halfway. Divide between plates and serve.

368.Snapper Fillets With Nutty Tomato Sauce

Servings: 4
Cooking Time: 20 Minutes
Ingredients:
- 4 skin-on snapper fillets
- Sea salt and ground pepper, to taste
- 1/2 cup parmesan cheese, grated
- 2 tablespoons fresh cilantro, chopped
- 1/2 cup coconut flour
- 2 tablespoon flaxseed meal
- 2 medium-sized eggs
- For the Almond sauce:
- 1/4 cup almonds
- 2 garlic cloves, pressed
- 1 cup tomato paste
- 1 teaspoon dried dill weed
- 1/2 teaspoon salt
- 1/4 teaspoon freshly ground mixed peppercorns
- 1/4 cup olive oil

Directions:
1. Season fish fillets with sea salt and pepper.
2. In a shallow plate, thoroughly combine the parmesan cheese and fresh chopped cilantro.
3. In another shallow plate, whisk the eggs until frothy. Place the coconut flour and flaxseed meal in a third plate.
4. Dip the fish fillets in the flour, then in the egg; afterward, coat them with the parmesan mixture. Set the Air Fryer to cook at 390 degrees F; air fry for 14 to 16 minutes or until crisp.
5. To make the sauce, chop the almonds in a food processor. Add the remaining sauce ingredients, but not the olive oil.
6. Blitz for 30 seconds; then, slowly and gradually pour in the oil; process until smooth and even. Serve the sauce with the prepared snapper fillets. Bon appétit!

369.Favorite Shrimp Fritatta

Servings:4
Cooking Time: 25 Minutes
Ingredients:
- Pinch salt
- ½ cup rice, cooked
- ½ cup baby spinach
- ½ cup Monterey Jack cheese, grated
- ½ cup shrimp, chopped and cooked

Directions:
1. Preheat air fryer to 320 F. In a bowl, add eggs, salt, and basil; stir until frothy. Spray baking pan with cooking spray. Add in rice, spinach and shrimp. Pour egg mixture over and top with cheese. Place the pan in the air fryer's basket and cook for 14 minutes until the frittata is puffed and golden brown. Serve.

370.Cheese Crust Salmon

Servings: 5
Cooking Time: 20 Minutes
Ingredients:
- 2 lb. salmon fillet
- 2 garlic cloves, minced
- ¼ cup fresh parsley, chopped
- ½ cup parmesan cheese, grated
- Salt and pepper to taste

Directions:
1. Pre-heat the Air Fryer to 350°F.
2. Lay the salmon, skin-side-down, on a sheet of aluminum foil. Place another sheet of foil on top.
3. Transfer the salmon to the fryer and cook for 10 minutes.
4. Remove the salmon from the fryer. Take off the top layer of foil and add the minced garlic, parmesan cheese, pepper, salt and parsley on top of the fish.
5. Return the salmon to the Air Fryer and resume cooking for another minute.

371.Buttered Baked Cod With Wine

Servings:2
Cooking Time: 12 Minutes
Ingredients:
- 1 tablespoon butter
- 1 tablespoon butter

- 2 tablespoons dry white wine
- 1/2 pound thick-cut cod loin
- 1-1/2 teaspoons chopped fresh parsley
- 1-1/2 teaspoons chopped green onion
- 1/2 lemon, cut into wedges
- 1/4 sleeve buttery round crackers (such as Ritz®), crushed
- 1/4 lemon, juiced

Directions:
1. In a small bowl, melt butter in microwave. Whisk in crackers.
2. Lightly grease baking pan of air fryer with remaining butter. And melt for 2 minutes at 390 °F.
3. In a small bowl whisk well lemon juice, white wine, parsley, and green onion.
4. Coat cod filets in melted butter. Pour dressing. Top with butter-cracker mixture.
5. Cook for 10 minutes at 390 °F.
6. Serve and enjoy with a slice of lemon.

372.Air Fried Catfish

Servings: 4
Cooking Time: 20 Minutes
Ingredients:
- 4 catfish fillets
- 1 tbsp olive oil
- 1/4 cup fish seasoning
- 1 tbsp fresh parsley, chopped

Directions:
1. Preheat the air fryer to 400 F.
2. Spray air fryer basket with cooking spray.
3. Seasoned fish with seasoning and place into the air fryer basket.
4. Drizzle fish fillets with oil and cook for 10 minutes.
5. Turn fish to another side and cook for 10 minutes more.
6. Garnish with parsley and serve.

373.Jamaican-style Fish And Potato Fritters

Servings: 2
Cooking Time: 30 Minutes
Ingredients:
- 1/2 pound sole fillets
- 1/2 pound mashed potatoes
- 1 egg, well beaten
- 1/2 cup red onion, chopped
- 2 garlic cloves, minced
- 2 tablespoons fresh parsley, chopped
- 1 bell pepper, finely chopped
- 1/2 teaspoon scotch bonnet pepper, minced
- 1 tablespoon olive oil
- 1 tablespoon coconut aminos
- 1/2 teaspoon paprika
- Salt and white pepper, to taste

Directions:

1. Start by preheating your Air Fryer to 395 degrees F. Spritz the sides and bottom of the cooking basket with cooking spray.
2. Cook the sole fillets in the preheated Air Fryer for 10 minutes, flipping them halfway through the cooking time.
3. In a mixing bowl, mash the sole fillets into flakes. Stir in the remaining ingredients. Shape the fish mixture into patties.
4. Bake in the preheated Air Fryer at 390 degrees F for 14 minutes, flipping them halfway through the cooking time. Bon appétit!

374.Lobster Tails With Olives And Butter

Servings: 5
Cooking Time: 20 Minutes
Ingredients:
- 2 pounds fresh lobster tails, cleaned and halved, in shells
- 2 tablespoons butter, melted
- 1 teaspoon onion powder
- 1 teaspoon cayenne pepper
- Salt and ground black pepper, to taste
- 2 garlic cloves, minced
- 1 cup green olives

Directions:
1. In a plastic closeable bag, thoroughly combine all ingredients; shake to combine well.
2. Transfer the coated lobster tails to the greased cooking basket.
3. Cook in the preheated Air Fryer at 390 degrees for 6 to 7 minutes, shaking the basket halfway through. Work in batches.
4. Serve with green olives and enjoy!

375.Outrageous Crispy Fried Salmon Skin

Servings:4
Cooking Time: 10 Minutes
Ingredients:
- ½ pound salmon skin, patted dry
- 4 tablespoons coconut oil
- Salt and pepper to taste

Directions:
1. Preheat the air fryer for 5 minutes.
2. In a large bowl, combine everything and mix well.
3. Place in the fryer basket and close.
4. Cook for 10 minutes at 400°F.
5. Halfway through the cooking time, give a good shake to evenly cook the skin.

376.Tilapia And Tomato Salsa

Servings: 4
Cooking Time: 15 Minutes
Ingredients:
- 4 tilapia fillets, boneless
- 1 tablespoon olive oil

- A pinch of salt and black pepper
- 12 ounces tomatoes, chopped
- 2 tablespoons green onions, chopped
- 2 tablespoons sweet red pepper, chopped
- 1 tablespoon balsamic vinegar

Directions:
1. Arrange the tilapia in a baking sheet that fits the air fryer and season with salt and pepper. In a bowl, combine all the other ingredients, toss and spread over the fish. Introduce the pan in the fryer and cook at 350 degrees F for 15 minutes. Divide the mix between plates and serve.

377.Creole Crab

Servings: 6
Cooking Time: 6 Minutes
Ingredients:
- 1 teaspoon Creole seasonings
- 4 tablespoons almond flour
- ¼ teaspoon baking powder
- 1 teaspoon apple cider vinegar
- ¼ teaspoon onion powder
- 1 teaspoon dried dill
- 1 teaspoon ghee
- 13 oz crab meat, finely chopped
- 1 egg, beaten
- Cooking spray

Directions:
1. In the mixing bowl mix up crab meat, egg, dried dill, ghee, onion powder, apple cider vinegar, baking powder, and Creole seasonings. Then add almond flour and stir the mixture with the help of the fork until it is homogenous. Make the small balls (hushpuppies). Preheat the air fryer to 390F. Put the hushpuppies in the air fryer basket and spray with cooking spray. Cook them for 3 minutes. Then flip them on another side and cook for 3 minutes more or until the hushpuppies are golden brown.

378.Grilled Fish And Celery Burgers

Servings: 4
Cooking Time: 10 Minutes + Chilling Time
Ingredients:
- 2 cans canned tuna fish
- 2 celery stalks, trimmed and finely chopped
- 1 egg, whisked
- 1/2 cup parmesan cheese, grated
- 1 teaspoon whole-grain mustard
- 1/2 teaspoon sea salt
- 1/4 teaspoon freshly cracked black peppercorns
- 1 teaspoon paprika

Directions:
1. Mix all of the above ingredients in the order listed above; mix to combine well and shape into four cakes; chill for 50 minutes.

2. Place on an Air Fryer grill pan. Spritz each cake with a non-stick cooking spray, covering all sides.
3. Grill at 360 degrees F for 5 minutes; then, pause the machine, flip the cakes over and set the timer for another 3 minutes. Serve over mashed potatoes.

379.Creamy Tilapia

Servings: 2
Cooking Time: 12 Minutes
Ingredients:
- 8 oz tilapia fillet
- 1 teaspoon coconut cream
- 1 teaspoon coconut flour
- ½ teaspoon salt
- ¼ teaspoon smoked paprika
- ½ teaspoon dried oregano
- ½ teaspoon coconut oil, melted
- ¼ teaspoon ground cumin

Directions:
1. Rub the tilapia fillet with ground cumin, dried oregano, smoked paprika, and salt. Then dip it in the coconut cream. Cut the tilapia fillet on 2 servings. After this, sprinkle every tilapia fillet with coconut flour gently. Preheat the air fryer to 385F. Sprinkle the air fryer basket with coconut oil and put the tilapia fillets inside. Cook the fillets for 6 minutes from every side.

380.Beer Battered Fish With Honey Tartar Sauce

Servings: 2
Cooking Time: 20 Minutes
Ingredients:
- 1/2 pound hoki fillets
- Sea salt and black pepper, to taste
- 1/2 cup flour
- 1 egg
- 1 teaspoon paprika
- 1 (12-ounce) bottle beer
- 1/4 cup mayonnaise
- 1/2 teaspoon honey
- 1 tablespoon fresh lemon juice
- 1 teaspoon Dijon mustard
- 1 teaspoon sweet pickle relish

Directions:
1. Rinse the hoki fillets and pat dry.
2. Combine the flour, egg and paprika in a bowl. Gradually pour in beer until a batter is formed.
3. Dip the fish fillets into the batter; then, transfer to the lightly greased cooking basket. Cook in the preheated Air Fryer at 380 degrees F for 12 minutes.
4. In the meantime, whisk the remaining ingredients to make the sauce. Place in the

96

refrigerator until ready to serve. Bon
appétit!

381.Paprika Tilapia

Servings: 4
Cooking Time: 20 Minutes
Ingredients:
- 4 tilapia fillets, boneless
- 3 tablespoons ghee, melted
- A pinch of salt and black pepper
- 2 tablespoons capers
- 1 teaspoon garlic powder
- ½ teaspoon smoked paprika
- ½ teaspoon oregano, dried
- 2 tablespoons lemon juice

Directions:
1. In a bowl, mix all the ingredients except the
   fish and toss. Arrange the fish in a pan that
   fits the air fryer, pour the capers mix all
   over, put the pan in the air fryer and cook
   360 degrees F for 20 minutes, shaking
   halfway. Divide between plates and serve
   hot.

382.King Prawns With Lemon Butter Sauce

Servings: 4
Cooking Time: 15 Minutes
Ingredients:
- King Prawns:
- 1 ½ pounds king prawns, peeled and
  deveined
- 2 cloves garlic, minced
- 1/2 cup Pecorino Romano cheese, grated
- Sea salt and ground white pepper, to your
  liking
- 1/2 teaspoon onion powder
- 1 teaspoon garlic powder
- 1 teaspoon mustard seeds
- 2 tablespoons olive oil
- Sauce:
- 2 tablespoons butter
- 2 tablespoons fresh lemon juice
- 1/2 teaspoon Worcestershire sauce
- 1/4 teaspoon ground black pepper

Directions:
1. In a plastic closeable bag, thoroughly
   combine all ingredients for the king prawns;
   shake to combine well.
2. Transfer the coated king prawns to the
   lightly greased Air Fryer basket.
3. Cook in the preheated Air Fryer at 390
   degrees for 6 minutes, shaking the basket
   halfway through. Work in batches.
4. In the meantime, heat a small saucepan
   over a moderate flame; melt the butter and
   add the remaining ingredients.
5. Turn the temperature to low and whisk for
   2 to 3 minutes until thoroughly heated.

Spoon the sauce onto the warm king
prawns. Bon appétit!

383.Parmesan And Garlic Trout

Servings: 4
Cooking Time: 15 Minutes
Ingredients:
- 2 tablespoons olive oil
- 2 garlic cloves, minced
- ½ cup chicken stock
- Salt and black pepper to the taste
- 4 trout fillets, boneless
- ¾ cup parmesan, grated
- ¼ cup tarragon, chopped

Directions:
1. In a pan that fits your air fryer, mix all the
   ingredients except the fish and the
   parmesan and whisk. Add the fish and
   grease it well with this mix. Sprinkle the
   parmesan on top, put the pan in the air
   fryer and cook at 380 degrees F for 15
   minutes. Divide everything between plates
   and serve.

384.Hake Fillets With Classic Garlic Sauce

Servings: 3
Cooking Time: 20 Minutes
Ingredients:
- 3 hake fillets
- 6 tablespoons mayonnaise
- 1 teaspoon Dijon mustard
- 1 tablespoon fresh lime juice
- 1 cup parmesan cheese, grated
- Salt, to taste
- 1/4 teaspoon ground black pepper, or more
  to taste
- Garlic Sauce
- 1/4 cup Greek-style yogurt
- 2 tablespoons olive oil
- 2 cloves garlic, minced
- 1/2 teaspoon tarragon leaves, minced

Directions:
1. Pat dry the hake fillets with a kitchen towel.
2. In a shallow bowl, whisk together the
   mayonnaise, mustard, and lime juice. In
   another shallow bowl, thoroughly combine
   the parmesan cheese with salt, and black
   pepper.
3. Dip the fish fillets in the mayo mixture; then,
   press them over the parmesan mixture.
4. Spritz the Air Fryer grill pan with non-stick
   cooking spray. Grill in the preheated Air Fry
   at 395 degrees F for 10 minutes, flipping
   halfway through the cooking time.
5. Meanwhile, make the sauce by whisking all
   the ingredients. Serve warm fish fillets with
   the sauce on the side. Bon appétit!

385.Air Fried Fresh Broiled Tilapia

Servings:4
Cooking Time: 15 Minutes
Ingredients:
- 1 tbsp old bay seasoning
- 2 tbsp canola oil
- 2 tbsp lemon pepper
- Salt to taste
- 2-3 butter buds

Directions:
1. Preheat fryer to 400 F. Drizzle oil over tilapia. In a bowl, mix salt, lemon pepper, butter buds, and seasoning; spread on the fish. Place the fillets in the air fryer and cook for 10 minutes until crispy.

386.Quick And Easy Shrimp

Servings:2
Cooking Time:5 Minutes
Ingredients:
- ½ pound tiger shrimp
- 1 tablespoon olive oil
- ½ teaspoon old bay seasoning
- ¼ teaspoon smoked paprika
- ¼ teaspoon cayenne pepper
- Salt, to taste

Directions:
1. Preheat the Air fryer to 390 °F and grease an Air fryer basket.
2. Mix all the ingredients in a large bowl until well combined.
3. Place the shrimps in the Air fryer basket and cook for about 5 minutes.
4. Dish out and serve warm.

387.Paprika Snapper Mix

Servings: 4
Cooking Time: 14 Minutes
Ingredients:
- 4 snapper fillets, boneless and skin scored
- 2 tablespoons sweet paprika
- 3 tablespoons olive oil
- A pinch of salt and black pepper
- 6 spring onions, chopped
- Juice of ½ lemon

Directions:
1. In a bowl, mix the paprika with the rest of the ingredients except the fish and whisk well. Rub the fish with this mix, place the fillets in your air fryer's basket and cook at 390 degrees F for 7 minutes on each side. Divide between plates and serve with a side salad.

388.Greek-style Salmon With Dill Sauce

Servings:4
Cooking Time: 25 Minutes
Ingredients:
- Salt and pepper to taste
- 2 tsp olive oil
- 3 tbsp chopped dill + extra for garnishing
- 1 cup sour cream
- 1 cup Greek yogurt

Directions:
1. For the dill sauce, in a bowl, mix well the sour cream, yogurt, dill, and salt. Preheat air fryer to 280 F.
2. Drizzle the olive oil over the salmon, and rub with salt and pepper. Arrange the salmon pieces in the fryer basket and cook them for 15 minutes. Remove salmon to a platter and top with the sauce. Serve.

389.Paprika Cod And Endives

Servings: 4
Cooking Time: 20 Minutes
Ingredients:
- 2 endives, shredded
- 2 tablespoons olive oil
- Salt and back pepper to the taste
- 4 salmon fillets, boneless
- ½ teaspoon sweet paprika

Directions:
1. In a pan that fits the air fryer, combine the fish with the rest of the ingredients, toss, introduce in the fryer and cook at 350 degrees F for 20 minutes, flipping the fish halfway. Divide between plates and serve right away.

390.Tuna Skewers

Servings: 4
Cooking Time: 12 Minutes
Ingredients:
- 1 pound tuna steaks, boneless and cubed
- 1 chili pepper, minced
- 4 green onions, chopped
- 2 tablespoons lime juice
- A drizzle of olive oil
- Salt and black pepper to the taste

Directions:
1. In a bowl mix all the ingredients and toss them. Thread the tuna cubes on skewers, arrange them in your air fryer's basket and cook at 370 degrees F for 12 minutes. Divide between plates and serve with a side salad.

391.Crusted Flounder Fillets

Servings: 2
Cooking Time: 20 Minutes
Ingredients:
- 2 flounder fillets
- 1 egg
- 1/2 teaspoon Worcestershire sauce
- 1/4 cup coconut flour
- 1/4 cup almond flour
- 1/2 teaspoon lemon pepper

- 1/2 teaspoon coarse sea salt
- 1/4 teaspoon chili powder

Directions:
1. Rinse and pat dry the flounder fillets.
2. Whisk the egg and Worcestershire sauce in a shallow bowl. In a separate bowl, mix the coconut flour, almond flour, lemon pepper, salt, and chili powder.
3. Then, dip the fillets into the egg mixture. Lastly, coat the fish fillets with the coconut flour mixture until they are coated on all sides.
4. Spritz with cooking spray and transfer to the Air Fryer basket. Cook at 390 degrees for 7 minutes.
5. Turn them over, spritz with cooking spray on the other side, and cook another 5 minutes. Bon appétit!

392.Minty Trout And Pine Nuts

Servings: 4
Cooking Time: 16 Minutes
Ingredients:
- 4 rainbow trout
- 1 cup olive oil + 3 tablespoons
- Juice of 1 lemon
- A pinch of salt and black pepper
- 1 cup parsley, chopped
- 3 garlic cloves, minced
- ½ cup mint, chopped
- Zest of 1 lemon
- 1/3 pine nuts
- 1 avocado, peeled, pitted and roughly chopped

Directions:
1. Pat dry the trout, season with salt and pepper and rub with 3 tablespoons oil. Put the fish in your air fryer's basket and cook for 8 minutes on each side. Divide the fish between plates and drizzle half of the lemon juice all over. In a blender, combine the rest of the oil with the remaining lemon juice, parsley, garlic, mint, lemon zest, pine nuts and the avocado and pulse well. Spread this over the trout and serve.

393.Cajun-rubbed Jumbo Shrimp

Servings:2
Cooking Time: 10 Minutes
Ingredients:
- Salt to taste
- ¼ tsp old bay seasoning
- ⅓ tsp smoked paprika
- ¼ tsp cayenne pepper
- 1 tbsp olive oil

Directions:
1. Preheat air fryer to 390 degrees. In a bowl, add shrimp, paprika, oil, salt, old bay seasoning, and cayenne pepper; mix well.

Place the shrimp in the fryer and cook for 5 minutes. Serve with aioli.

394.Crisped Flounder Filet With Crumb Tops

Servings:4
Cooking Time: 15 Minutes
Ingredients:
- 1 cup dry bread crumbs
- 1 egg beaten
- 1 lemon, sliced
- 4 pieces of flounder fillets
- 5 tablespoons vegetable oil

Directions:
1. Brush flounder fillets with vegetable oil before dredging in bread crumbs.
2. Preheat the air fryer to 390°F.
3. Place the fillets on the double layer rack.
4. Cook for 15 minutes.

395.Char-grilled 'n Herbed Sea Scallops

Servings:3
Cooking Time: 10 Minutes
Ingredients:
- 1-pound sea scallops, meat only
- 3 tablespoons olive oil, divided
- 1 teaspoon dried sage
- Salt and pepper to taste
- 1 cup grape tomatoes, halved
- 1/3 cup basil leaves, shredded

Directions:
1. Preheat the air fryer at 390°F.
2. Place the grill pan accessory in the air fryer.
3. Season the scallops with half of the olive oil, sage, salt and pepper.
4. Toss into the air fryer and grill for 10 minutes.
5. Once cooked, serve with tomatoes and basil leaves.
6. Drizzle the remaining olive oil and season with more salt and pepper to taste.

396.Shrimp And Pine Nuts Mix

Servings: 4
Cooking Time: 12 Minutes
Ingredients:
- ½ cup parsley leaves
- ½ cup basil leaves
- 2 tablespoons lemon juice
- 1/3 cup pine nuts
- ¼ cup parmesan, grated
- A pinch of salt and black pepper
- ½ cup olive oil
- 1 and ½ pounds shrimp, peeled and deveined
- ¼ teaspoon lemon zest, grated

Directions:
1. In a blender, combine all the ingredients except the shrimp and pulse well. In a bowl,

mix the shrimp with the pesto and toss. Put the shrimp in your air fryer's basket and cook at 360 degrees F for 12 minutes, flipping the shrimp halfway. Divide the shrimp into bowls and serve.

397.Steamed Salmon With Dill Sauce

Servings:2
Cooking Time:11 Minutes
Ingredients:
- 1 cup water
- 2 (6-ounce) salmon fillets
- ½ cup Greek yogurt
- 2 tablespoons fresh dill, chopped and divided
- 2 teaspoons olive oil
- Salt, to taste
- ½ cup sour cream

Directions:
1. Preheat the Air fryer to 285 °F and grease an Air fryer basket.
2. Place water the bottom of the Air fryer pan.
3. Coat salmon with olive oil and season with a pinch of salt.
4. Arrange the salmon in the Air fryer and cook for about 11 minutes.
5. Meanwhile, mix remaining ingredients in a bowl to make dill sauce.
6. Serve the salmon with dill sauce.

398.Spiced Catfish

Servings:4
Cooking Time:23 Minutes
Ingredients:
- 4 (6-ounces) catfish fillets
- 1 tablespoon olive oil
- 2 tablespoons corn meal
- 2 tablespoons corn flour
- 2 tablespoons garlic
- 2 tablespoons salt

Directions:
1. Preheat the Air fryer to 400 °F and grease an Air fryer basket.
2. Mix the catfish fillets with corn meal, corn flour, garlic and salt in a bowl.
3. Drizzle with olive oil and arrange catfish fillets into the Air fryer basket.
4. Cook for about 10 minutes and flip the side.
5. Cook for another 10 minutes and flip again.
6. Cook for about 3 more minutes and dish out the catfish fillets to serve hot.

399.Tuna Patties With Cheese Sauce

Servings: 4
Cooking Time: 2 Hours 20 Minutes
Ingredients:
- 1 pound canned tuna, drained
- 1 egg, whisked
- 1 garlic clove, minced

- 2 tablespoons shallots, minced
- 1 cup Romano cheese, grated
- Sea salt and ground black pepper, to taste
- 1 tablespoon sesame oil
- Cheese Sauce:
- 1 tablespoon butter
- 1 cup beer
- 2 tablespoons Colby cheese, grated

Directions:
1. In a mixing bowl, thoroughly combine the tuna, egg, garlic, shallots, Romano cheese, salt, and black pepper. Shape the tuna mixture into four patties and place in your refrigerator for 2 hours.
2. Brush the patties with sesame oil on both sides. Cook in the preheated Air Fryer at 360 degrees F for 14 minutes.
3. In the meantime, melt the butter in a pan over a moderate heat. Add the beer and whisk until it starts bubbling.
4. Now, stir in the grated cheese and cook for 3 to 4 minutes longer or until the cheese has melted. Spoon the sauce over the fish cake burgers and serve immediately.

400.Flavored Jamaican Salmon Recipe

Servings: 4
Cooking Time:20 Minutes
Ingredients:
- 4 cups baby arugula
- 2 cups radish; julienned
- 2 tsp. sriracha sauce
- 4 tsp. sugar
- 3 scallions; chopped
- 2 cups cabbage; shredded
- 1 ½ tsp. Jamaican jerk seasoning
- 1/4 cup pepitas; toasted
- 2 tsp. olive oil
- 4 tsp. apple cider vinegar
- 3 tsp. avocado oil
- 4 medium salmon fillets; boneless
- Salt and black pepper to the taste

Directions:
1. In a bowl; mix sriracha with sugar, whisk and transfer 2 tsp. to another bowl.
2. Combine 2 tsp. sriracha mix with the avocado oil, olive oil, vinegar, salt and pepper and whisk well.
3. Sprinkle jerk seasoning over salmon, rub with sriracha and sugar mix and season with salt and pepper.
4. Transfer to your air fryer and cook at 360 °F, for 10 minutes; flipping once.
5. In a bowl; mix radishes with cabbage, arugula, salt, pepper, sriracha and vinegar mix and toss well. Divide salmon and radish mix on plates, sprinkle pepitas and scallions on top and serve.

401.Mahi Mahi And Broccoli Cakes

Servings: 4
Cooking Time: 11 Minutes
Ingredients:
- ½ cup broccoli, shredded
- 1 tablespoon flax meal
- 1 egg, beaten
- 1 teaspoon ground coriander
- 1 oz Monterey Jack cheese, shredded
- ½ teaspoon salt
- 6 oz Mahi Mahi, chopped
- Cooking spray

Directions:
1. In the mixing bowl mix up flax meal, egg, ground coriander, salt, broccoli, and chopped Mahi Mahi. Stir the ingredients gently with the help of the fork and add shredded Monterey Jack cheese. Stir the mixture until homogenous. Then make 4 cakes. Preheat the air fryer to 390F. Place the Mahi Mahi cakes in the air fryer and spray them gently with cooking spray. Cook the fish cakes for 5 minutes and then flip on another side. Cook the fish cakes for 6 minutes more.

402.Cajun Cod Fillets With Avocado Sauce

Servings: 2
Cooking Time: 20 Minutes
Ingredients:
- 2 cod fish fillets
- 1 egg
- Sea salt, to taste
- 1/2 cup tortilla chips, crushed
- 2 teaspoons olive oil
- 1/2 avocado, peeled, pitted, and mashed
- 1 tablespoon mayonnaise
- 3 tablespoons sour cream
- 1/2 teaspoon yellow mustard
- 1 teaspoon lemon juice
- 1 garlic clove, minced
- 1/4 teaspoon black pepper
- 1/4 teaspoon salt
- 1/4 teaspoon hot pepper sauce

Directions:
1. Start by preheating your Air Fryer to 360 degrees F. Spritz the Air Fryer basket with cooking oil.
2. Pat dry the fish fillets with a kitchen towel. Beat the egg in a shallow bowl.
3. In a separate bowl, thoroughly combine the salt, crushed tortilla chips, and olive oil.
4. Dip the fish into the egg, then, into the crumb mixture, making sure to coat thoroughly. Cook in the preheated Air Fryer approximately 12 minutes.
5. Meanwhile, make the avocado sauce by mixing the remaining ingredients in a bowl.

Place in your refrigerator until ready to serve.
6. Serve the fish fillets with chilled avocado sauce on the side. Bon appétit!

403.Cod

Servings: 5
Cooking Time: 20 Minutes
Ingredients:
- 1 lb. cod
- 3 tbsp. milk
- 1 cup meal
- 2 cups friendly bread crumbs
- 2 large eggs, beaten
- ½ tsp. pepper
- ¼ tsp. salt

Directions:
1. Combine together the milk and eggs in a bowl.
2. In a shallow dish, stir together bread crumbs, pepper, and salt.
3. Pour the meal into a second shallow dish.
4. Coat the cod sticks with the meal before dipping each one in the egg and rolling in bread crumbs.
5. Put the fish sticks in the Air Fryer basket. Cook at 350°F for 12 minutes, shaking the basket halfway through cooking.

404.Old Bay Seasoned Shrimp

Servings:6
Cooking Time: 15 Minutes
Ingredients:
- ¼ tsp cayenne pepper
- ½ tsp old bay seasoning
- ¼ tsp smoked paprika
- A pinch of salt
- 1 tbsp olive oil

Directions:
1. Preheat your air fryer to 390 F, and in a bowl, mix all listed ingredients. Place the mixture in your air fryer's cooking basket and cook for 5 minutes. Serve with warm rice and a drizzle of lemon juice.

405.Char And Fennel

Servings: 4
Cooking Time: 18 Minutes
Ingredients:
- 4 char fillets, boneless
- 3 tablespoons olive oil
- 1 fennel bulb, sliced with a mandolin
- A pinch of salt and black pepper
- 5 garlic cloves, minced
- 1 teaspoon caraway seeds
- 2 tablespoons balsamic vinegar
- 1 tablespoon lemon juice
- 1 tablespoon lemon peel, grated
- ½ cup dill, chopped

Directions:

1. In a pan that fits your air fryer, mix the fish with all the other ingredients, toss, introduce in the air fryer and cook at 390 degrees F for 18 minutes. Divide the fish between plates and serve with a side salad.

406.Fish Fingers With Dijon Mayo Sauce

Servings: 4
Cooking Time: 15 Minutes
Ingredients:

- For the Fish:
- 1 pound white fish, cut into strips
- 1 ½ tablespoons olive oil
- 1/2 teaspoon garlic salt
- 1 teaspoon red pepper flakes, crushed
- 1/2 teaspoon dried dill weed
- 1/2 cup coconut flour
- 1/2 cup parmesan cheese, grated
- 2 medium-sized eggs, well whisked
- For the Dijon Sauce:
- 1 ½ tablespoons Dijon mustard
- 1/2 cup mayonnaise
- 1/2 teaspoon lemon juice, freshly squeezed

Directions:

1. Rub the fish strips with olive oil, salt, red pepper and dill weed. Then, prepare three shallow bowls.
2. Put the coconut flour into the first bowl. In another shallow bowl, place the eggs; in the third one, the parmesan cheese.
3. Meanwhile, preheat your machine to cook at 385 degrees F. Cover the fish strips with the coconut flour, and then with the eggs; finally, roll each fish piece over the parmesan cheese.
4. Air-fry for 5 minutes, then pause the machine, flip them over and cook for another 5 minutes or until cooked through.
5. In the meantime, make the sauce by mixing together all the sauce ingredients. Serve as a dipping sauce and enjoy!

407.Tarragon Sea Bass And Risotto

Servings: 4
Cooking Time: 25 Minutes
Ingredients:

- 4 sea bass fillets, boneless
- A pinch of salt and black pepper
- 1 tablespoon ghee, melted
- 1 garlic clove, minced
- 1 cup cauliflower rice
- ½ cup chicken stock
- 1 tablespoon parmesan, grated
- 1 tablespoon chervil, chopped
- 1 tablespoon parsley, chopped
- 1 tablespoon tarragon, chopped

Directions:

1. In a pan that fits your air fryer, mix the cauliflower rice with the stock, parmesan, chervil, tarragon and parsley, toss, introduce the pan in the air fryer and cook at 380 degrees F for 12 minutes. In a bowl, mix the fish with salt, pepper, garlic and melted ghee and toss gently. Put the fish over the cauliflower rice, cook at 380 degrees F for 12 minutes more, divide everything between plates and serve.

408.Sunday Fish With Sticky Sauce

Servings: 2
Cooking Time: 20 Minutes
Ingredients:

- 2 pollack fillets
- Salt and black pepper, to taste
- 1 tablespoon olive oil
- 1 cup chicken broth
- 2 tablespoons light soy sauce
- 1 tablespoon brown sugar
- 2 tablespoons butter, melted
- 1 teaspoon fresh ginger, minced
- 1 teaspoon fresh garlic, minced
- 2 corn tortillas

Directions:

1. Pat dry the pollack fillets and season them with salt and black pepper; drizzle the sesame oil all over the fish fillets.
2. Preheat the Air Fryer to 380 degrees F and cook your fish for 11 minutes. Slice into bite-sized pieces.
3. Meanwhile, prepare the sauce. Add the broth to a large saucepan and bring to a boil. Add the soy sauce, sugar, butter, ginger, and garlic. Reduce the heat to simmer and cook until it is reduced slightly.
4. Add the fish pieces to the warm sauce. Serve on corn tortillas and enjoy!

409.Easy Creamy Shrimp Nachos

Servings: 4
Cooking Time: 15 Minutes
Ingredients:

- 1 pound shrimp, cleaned and deveined
- 1 tablespoon olive oil
- 2 tablespoons fresh lemon juice
- 1 teaspoon paprika
- 1/4 teaspoon cumin powder
- 1/2 teaspoon shallot powder
- 1/2 teaspoon garlic powder
- Coarse sea salt and ground black pepper, to taste
- 1 (9-ounce bag corn tortilla chips
- 1/4 cup pickled jalapeño, minced
- 1 cup Pepper Jack cheese, grated
- 1/2 cup sour cream

Directions:

1. Toss the shrimp with the olive oil, lemon juice, paprika, cumin powder, shallot powder, garlic powder, salt, and black pepper.
2. Cook in the preheated Air Fryer at 390 degrees F for 5 minutes.
3. Place the tortilla chips on the aluminum foil-lined cooking basket. Top with the shrimp mixture, jalapeño and cheese. Cook another 2 minutes or until cheese has melted.
4. Serve garnished with sour cream and enjoy!

410.Salmon With Asparagus

Servings:2
Cooking Time: 11 Minutes
Ingredients:
- 2 (6-ounces) boneless salmon fillets
- 1½ tablespoons fresh lemon juice
- 1 tablespoon olive oil
- 2 tablespoons fresh parsley, roughly chopped
- 2 tablespoons fresh dill, roughly chopped
- 1 bunch asparagus
- Salt and ground black pepper, as required

Directions:
1. In a small bowl, mix well the lemon juice, oil, herbs, salt, and black pepper.
2. In another large bowl, mix together the salmon and ¾ of oil mixture.
3. In a second large bowl, add the asparagus and remaining oil mixture. Mix them well.
4. Set the temperature of air fryer to 400 degrees F. Grease an air fryer basket.
5. Arrange asparagus into the prepared air fryer basket.
6. Air fry for about 2-3 minutes.
7. Now, place the salmon fillets on top of asparagus and air fry for about 8 minutes.
8. Remove from air fryer and place the salmon fillets onto serving plates.
9. Serve hot alongside the asparagus.

411.Cajun Spiced Veggie-shrimp Bake

Servings:4
Cooking Time: 20 Minutes
Ingredients:
- 1 Bag of Frozen Mixed Vegetables
- 1 Tbsp Gluten Free Cajun Seasoning
- Olive Oil Spray
- Season with salt and pepper
- Small Shrimp Peeled & Deveined (Regular Size Bag about 50-80 Small Shrimp)

Directions:
1. Lightly grease baking pan of air fryer with cooking spray. Add all Ingredients and toss well to coat. Season with pepper and salt, generously.

2. For 10 minutes, cook on 330 °F. Halfway through cooking time, stir.
3. Cook for 10 minutes at 330 °F.
4. Serve and enjoy.

412.Crispy Fish Fingers With Lemon-garlic Herbs

Servings:1
Cooking Time: 10 Minutes
Ingredients:
- ¼ teaspoon baking soda
- ½ pound fish, cut into fingers
- ½ teaspoon crushed black pepper
- ½ teaspoon red chili flakes
- ½ teaspoon salt
- ½ teaspoon turmeric powder
- 1 cup bread crumbs
- 1 teaspoon ginger garlic paste
- 2 eggs, beaten
- 2 tablespoons lemon juice
- 2 teaspoons corn flour
- 2 teaspoons garlic powder
- Oil for brushing

Directions:
1. Preheat the air fryer to 390°F.
2. Season the fish fingers with salt, lemon juice, turmeric powder, chili flakes, garlic powder, black pepper, and garlic paste. Add the corn flour, eggs, and baking soda.
3. Dredge the seasoned fish in breadcrumbs and brush with cooking oil.
4. Place on the double layer rack.
5. Cook for 10 minutes.

413.Turmeric Salmon

Servings: 2
Cooking Time: 7 Minutes
Ingredients:
- 8 oz salmon fillet
- 2 tablespoons coconut flakes
- 1 tablespoon coconut cream
- ½ teaspoon salt
- ½ teaspoon ground turmeric
- ½ teaspoon onion powder
- 1 teaspoon nut oil

Directions:
1. Cut the salmon fillet into halves and sprinkle with salt, ground turmeric, and onion powder. After this, dip the fish fillets in the coconut cream and coat in the coconut flakes. Sprinkle the salmon fillets with nut oil. Preheat the air fryer to 380F. Arrange the salmon fillets in the air fryer basket and cook for 7 minutes.

414.Aromatic Shrimp With Herbs

Servings: 4
Cooking Time: 40 Minutes
Ingredients:

- 1/2 tablespoon fresh basil leaves, chopped
- 1 ½ pounds shrimp, shelled and deveined
- 1 ½ tablespoons olive oil
- 3 cloves garlic, minced
- 1 teaspoon smoked cayenne pepper
- 1/2 teaspoon fresh mint, roughly chopped
- ½ teaspoon ginger, freshly grated
- 1 teaspoon sea salt

Directions:
1. Firstly, set your Air Fryer to cook at 395 degrees F.
2. In a mixing dish, combine all of the above items; toss until everything is well combined and let it stand for about 28 minutes.
3. Air-fry for 3 to 4 minutes. Bon appétit!

415.Breaded Hake

Servings:2
Cooking Time:12 Minutes
Ingredients:
- 1 egg
- 4 ounces breadcrumbs
- 4 (6-ounces) hake fillets
- 1 lemon, cut into wedges
- 2 tablespoons vegetable oil

Directions:
1. Preheat the Air fryer to 350 °F and grease an Air fryer basket.
2. Whisk the egg in a shallow bowl and mix breadcrumbs and oil in another bowl.
3. Dip hake fillets into the whisked egg and then, dredge in the breadcrumb mixture.
4. Arrange the hake fillets into the Air fryer basket in a single layer and cook for about 12 minutes.
5. Dish out the hake fillets onto serving plates and serve, garnished with lemon wedges.

416.Smoked Halibut And Eggs In Brioche

Servings: 4
Cooking Time: 25 Minutes
Ingredients:
- 4 brioche rolls
- 1 pound smoked halibut, chopped
- 4 eggs
- 1 teaspoon dried thyme
- 1 teaspoon dried basil
- Salt and black pepper, to taste

Directions:
1. Cut off the top of each brioche; then, scoop out the insides to make the shells.
2. Lay the prepared brioche shells in the lightly greased cooking basket.
3. Spritz with cooking oil; add the halibut. Crack an egg into each brioche shell; sprinkle with thyme, basil, salt, and black pepper.

4. Bake in the preheated Air Fryer at 325 degrees F for 20 minutes. Bon appétit!

417.Buttery Haddock And Parsley

Servings: 2
Cooking Time: 16 Minutes
Ingredients:
- 7 oz haddock fillet
- 2 tablespoons butter, melted
- 1 teaspoon minced garlic
- ½ teaspoon salt
- 1 teaspoon fresh parsley, chopped
- ½ teaspoon ground celery root

Directions:
1. Cut the fish fillet on 2 servings. In the shallow bowl mix up butter and minced garlic. Then add salt, celery root, and fresh parsley. After this, carefully brush the fish fillets with the butter mixture. Then wrap every fillet in the foil. Preheat the air fryer to 385F. Put the wrapped haddock fillets in the air fryer and cook for 16 minutes.

418.Breaded Salmon

Servings: 4
Cooking Time: 25 Minutes
Ingredients:
- 2 cups friendly bread crumbs
- 4 fillets of salmon
- 1 cup Swiss cheese, shredded
- 2 eggs, beaten

Directions:
1. 1 Pre-heat your Air Fryer to 390°F.
2. 2 Dredge the salmon fillets into the eggs. Add the Swiss cheese on top of each fillet.
3. 3 Coat all sides of the fish with bread crumbs. Put in an oven safe dish, transfer to the fryer, and cook for 20 minutes.

419.Herbed Trout Mix

Servings: 4
Cooking Time: 20 Minutes
Ingredients:
- 4 trout fillets, boneless and skinless
- 1 tablespoon lemon juice
- 2 tablespoons olive oil
- A pinch of salt and black pepper
- 1 bunch asparagus, trimmed
- 2 tablespoons ghee, melted
- ¼ cup mixed chives and tarragon

Directions:
1. Mix the asparagus with half of the oil, salt and pepper, put it in your air fryer's basket, cook at 380 degrees F for 6 minutes and divide between plates. In a bowl, mix the trout with salt, pepper, lemon juice, the rest of the oil and the herbes and toss, Put the fillets in your air fryer's basket and cook at 380 degrees F for 7 minutes on each side.

Divide the fish next to the asparagus, drizzle the melted ghee all over and serve.

420.Cornmeal 'n Old Bay Battered Fish

Servings:6
Cooking Time: 15 Minutes
Ingredients:
- ¼ cup flour
- ½ teaspoon garlic powder
- ¾ cup fine cornmeal
- 1 teaspoon paprika
- 2 teaspoons old bay seasoning
- 6 fish fillets cut in half
- Salt and pepper to taste

Directions:
1. Preheat the air fryer to 330°F.
2. Place the cornmeal, flour, and seasonings in a Ziploc bag.
3. Add the fish fillets and shake until the fish is covered in flour.
4. Place on the double layer rack and cook for 15 minutes.

421.Italian Shrimp

Servings: 4
Cooking Time: 12 Minutes
Ingredients:
- 1 pound shrimp, peeled and deveined
- A pinch of salt and black pepper
- 1 tablespoon sesame seeds, toasted
- ½ teaspoon Italian seasoning
- 1 tablespoon olive oil

Directions:
1. In a bowl, mix the shrimp with the rest of the ingredients and toss well. Put the shrimp in the air fryer's basket, cook at 370 degrees F for 12 minutes, divide into bowls and serve,

422.Cheesy Lemon Halibut

Servings: 2
Cooking Time: 20 Minutes
Ingredients:
- 1 lb. halibut fillet
- ½ cup butter
- 2 ½ tbsp. mayonnaise
- 2 ½ tbsp. lemon juice
- ¾ cup parmesan cheese, grated

Directions:
1. Pre-heat your fryer at 375°F.
2. Spritz the halibut fillets with cooking spray and season as desired.
3. Put the halibut in the fryer and cook for twelve minutes.
4. In the meantime, combine the butter, mayonnaise, and lemon juice in a bowl with a hand mixer. Ensure a creamy texture is achieved.
5. Stir in the grated parmesan.

6. When the halibut is ready, open the drawer and spread the butter over the fish with a butter knife. Allow to cook for a further two minutes, then serve hot.

423.Cod With Avocado Mayo Sauce

Servings: 2
Cooking Time: 20 Minutes
Ingredients:
- 2 cod fish fillets
- 1 egg
- Sea salt, to taste
- 2 teaspoons olive oil
- 1/2 avocado, peeled, pitted, and mashed
- 1 tablespoon mayonnaise
- 3 tablespoons sour cream
- 1/2 teaspoon yellow mustard
- 1 teaspoon lemon juice
- 1 garlic clove, minced
- 1/4 teaspoon black pepper
- 1/4 teaspoon salt
- 1/4 teaspoon hot pepper sauce

Directions:
1. Start by preheating your Air Fryer to 360 degrees F. Spritz the Air Fryer basket with cooking oil.
2. Pat dry the fish fillets with a kitchen towel. Beat the egg in a shallow bowl. Add in the salt and olive oil.
3. Dip the fish into the egg mixture, making sure to coat thoroughly. Cook in the preheated Air Fryer approximately 12 minutes.
4. Meanwhile, make the avocado sauce by mixing the remaining ingredients in a bowl. Place in your refrigerator until ready to serve.
5. Serve the fish fillets with chilled avocado sauce on the side. Bon appétit!

424.Cumin, Thyme 'n Oregano Herbed Shrimps

Servings:4
Cooking Time: 6 Minutes
Ingredients:
- ¼ teaspoon cayenne pepper
- ¼ teaspoon red chili flakes
- 1 teaspoon cumin
- 1 teaspoon oregano
- 1 teaspoon salt
- 1 teaspoon thyme
- 2 tablespoons coconut oil
- 2 teaspoons cilantro
- 2 teaspoons onion powder
- 2 teaspoons smoked paprika
- 20 jumbo shrimps, peeled and deveined

Directions:
1. Preheat the air fryer to 390°F.
2. Season the shrimps with all the Ingredients.

3. Place the seasoned shrimps in the double layer rack.
4. Cook for 6 minutes.

425.Butter Flounder Fillets

Servings: 4
Cooking Time: 20 Minutes
Ingredients:
- 4 flounder fillets, boneless
- A pinch of salt and black pepper
- 1 cup parmesan, grated
- 4 tablespoons butter, melted
- 2 tablespoons olive oil

Directions:
1. In a bowl, mix the parmesan with salt, pepper, butter and the oil and stir well. Arrange the fish in a pan that fits the air fryer, spread the parmesan mix all over, introduce in the fryer and cook at 400 degrees F for 20 minutes. Divide between plates and serve with a side salad.

426.Salmon Cakes

Servings:4
Cooking Time: 15 Minutes
Ingredients:
- 14 oz boiled and mashed potatoes
- 2 oz flour
- A handful of capers
- A handful of chopped parsley
- 1 tsp olive oil
- zest of 1 lemon

Directions:
1. Place the mashed potatoes in a large bowl and flake the salmon over. Stir in capers, parsley, and lemon zest. Shape small cakes out of the mixture. Dust them with flour and place in the fridge to set, for 1 hour. Preheat the air fryer to 350 F. Brush the olive oil over the basket's bottom and add the cakes. Cook for 7 minutes.

427.Creamy Salmon

Servings: 2
Cooking Time: 20 Minutes
Ingredients:
- ¾ lb. salmon, cut into 6 pieces
- ¼ cup yogurt
- 1 tbsp. olive oil
- 1 tbsp. dill, chopped
- 3 tbsp. sour cream
- Salt to taste

Directions:
1. 1 Sprinkle some salt on the salmon.
2. 2 Put the salmon slices in the Air Fryer basket and add in a drizzle of olive oil.
3. 3 Air fry the salmon at 285°F for 10 minutes.
4. 4 In the meantime, combine together the cream, dill, yogurt, and salt.
5. 5 Plate up the salmon and pour the creamy sauce over it. Serve hot.

SNACKS & APPETIZERS RECIPES

428.Crab And Chives Balls

Servings: 8
Cooking Time: 20 Minutes
Ingredients:
- ½ cup coconut cream
- 2 tablespoons chives, mined
- 1 egg, whisked
- 1 teaspoon mustard
- 1 teaspoon lemon juice
- 16 ounces lump crabmeat, chopped
- 2/3 cup almond meal
- A pinch of salt and black pepper
- Cooking spray

Directions:
1. In a bowl, mix all the ingredients except the cooking spray and stir well. Shape medium balls out of this mix, place them in the fryer and cook at 390 degrees F for 20 minutes. Serve as an appetizer.

429.Mexican-style Corn On The Cob With Bacon

Servings: 4
Cooking Time: 20 Minutes
Ingredients:
- 2 slices bacon
- 4 ears fresh corn, shucked and cut into halves
- 1 avocado, pitted, peeled and mashed
- 1 teaspoon ancho chili powder
- 2 garlic cloves
- 2 tablespoons cilantro, chopped
- 1 teaspoon lime juice
- Salt and black pepper, to taste

Directions:
1. Start by preheating your Air Fryer to 400 degrees F. Cook the bacon for 6 to 7 minutes; chop into small chunks and reserve.
2. Spritz the corn with cooking spray. Cook at 395 degrees F for 8 minutes, turning them over halfway through the cooking time.
3. Mix the reserved bacon with the remaining ingredients. Spoon the bacon mixture over the corn on the cob and serve immediately. Bon appétit!

430.Greek-style Squash Chips

Servings: 4
Cooking Time: 25 Minutes
Ingredients:
- 1/2 cup seasoned breadcrumbs
- 1/2 cup Parmesan cheese, grated
- Sea salt and ground black pepper, to taste
- 1/4 teaspoon oregano
- 2 yellow squash, cut into slices
- 2 tablespoons grapeseed oil

- Sauce:
- 1/2 cup Greek-style yogurt
- 1 tablespoon fresh cilantro, chopped
- 1 garlic clove, minced
- Freshly ground black pepper, to your liking

Directions:
1. In a shallow bowl, thoroughly combine the seasoned breadcrumbs, Parmesan, salt, black pepper, and oregano.
2. Dip the yellow squash slices in the prepared batter, pressing to adhere.
3. Brush with the grapeseed oil and cook in the preheated Air Fryer at 400 degrees F for 12 minutes. Shake the Air Fryer basket periodically to ensure even cooking. Work in batches.
4. While the chips are baking, whisk the sauce ingredients; place in your refrigerator until ready to serve. Enjoy!

431.Chives Meatballs

Servings: 6
Cooking Time: 20 Minutes
Ingredients:
- 1 pound beef meat, ground
- 1 teaspoon onion powder
- 1 teaspoon garlic powder
- A pinch of salt and black pepper
- 2 tablespoons chives, chopped
- Cooking spray

Directions:
1. In a bowl, mix all the ingredients except the cooking spray, stir well and shape medium meatballs out of this mix. Pace them in your lined air fryer's basket, grease with cooking spray and cook at 360 degrees F for 20 minutes. Serve as an appetizer.

432.Air Fried Chicken Tenders

Servings:4
Cooking Time:10 Minutes
Ingredients:
- 12 oz chicken breasts, cut into tenders
- 1 egg white
- 1/8 cup flour
- ½ cup panko bread crumbs
- Salt and black pepper, to taste

Directions:
1. Preheat the Air fryer to 350 °F and grease an Air fryer basket.
2. Season the chicken tenders with salt and black pepper.
3. Coat the chicken tenders with flour, then dip in egg whites and then dredge in the panko bread crumbs.
4. Arrange in the Air fryer basket and cook for about 10 minutes.

5. Dish out in a platter and serve warm.

433.Parmesan Turnip Slices

Servings: 8
Cooking Time: 10 Minutes
Ingredients:
- 1 lb turnip, peel and cut into slices
- 1 tbsp olive oil
- 3 oz parmesan cheese, shredded
- 1 tsp garlic powder
- 1 tsp salt

Directions:
1. Preheat the air fryer to 360 F.
2. Add all ingredients into the mixing bowl and toss to coat.
3. Transfer turnip slices into the air fryer basket and cook for 10 minutes.
4. Serve and enjoy.

434.Parsnip Chips With Spicy Citrus Aioli

Servings: 4
Cooking Time: 20 Minutes
Ingredients:
- 1 pound parsnips, peel long strips
- 2 tablespoons sesame oil
- Sea salt and ground black pepper, to taste
- 1 teaspoon red pepper flakes, crushed
- 1/2 teaspoon curry powder
- 1/2 teaspoon mustard seeds
- Spicy Citrus Aioli:
- 1/4 cup mayonnaise
- 1 tablespoon fresh lime juice
- 1 clove garlic, smashed
- Salt and black pepper, to taste

Directions:
1. Start by preheating the Air Fryer to 380 degrees F.
2. Toss the parsnip chips with the sesame oil, salt, black pepper, red pepper, curry powder, and mustard seeds.
3. Cook for 15 minutes, shaking the Air Fryer basket periodically.
4. Meanwhile, make the sauce by whisking the mayonnaise, lime juice, garlic, salt, and pepper. Place in the refrigerator until ready to use. Bon appétit!

435.Artichokes And Cream Cheese Dip

Servings: 6
Cooking Time: 25 Minutes
Ingredients:
- 2 teaspoons olive oil
- 2 spring onions, minced
- 1 pound artichoke hearts, steamed and chopped
- 2 garlic cloves, minced
- 6 ounces cream cheese, soft
- ½ cup almond milk
- 1 cup mozzarella, shredded

- A pinch of salt and black pepper

Directions:
1. Grease a baking pan that fits the air fryer with the oil and mix all the ingredients except the mozzarella inside. Sprinkle the cheese all over, introduce the pan in the air fryer and cook at 370 degrees F for 25 minutes. Divide into bowls and serve as a party dip.

436.Chicken Nuggets

Servings:4
Cooking Time:10 Minutes
Ingredients:
- 20-ounce chicken breast, cut into chunks
- 1 cup all-purpose flour
- 2 tablespoons milk
- 1 egg
- 1 cup panko breadcrumbs
- ½ tablespoon mustard powder
- 1 tablespoon garlic powder
- 1 tablespoon onion powder
- Salt and black pepper, to taste

Directions:
1. Preheat the Air fryer to 390 °F and grease an Air fryer basket.
2. Put chicken along with mustard powder, garlic powder, onion powder, salt and black pepper in a food processor and pulse until combined.
3. Place flour in a shallow dish and whisk the eggs with milk in a second dish.
4. Place breadcrumbs in a third shallow dish.
5. Coat the nuggets evenly in flour and dip in the egg mixture.
6. Roll into the breadcrumbs evenly and arrange the nuggets in an Air fryer basket.
7. Cook for about 10 minutes and dish out to serve warm.

437.Air Fried Cheese Sticks

Servings: 4 Minutes
Cooking Time: 8 Minutes
Ingredients:
- 6 mozzarella cheese sticks
- 1/4 tsp garlic powder
- 1 tsp Italian seasoning
- 1/3 cup almond flour
- 1/2 cup parmesan cheese, grated
- 1 large egg, lightly beaten
- 1/4 tsp sea salt

Directions:
1. In a small bowl, whisk the egg.
2. In a shallow bowl, mix together almond flour, parmesan cheese, Italian seasoning, garlic powder, and salt.
3. Dip mozzarella cheese stick in egg then coat with almond flour mixture and place on a plate. Place in refrigerator for1 hour.

4. Spray air fryer basket with cooking spray.
5. Place prepared mozzarella cheese sticks into the air fryer basket and cook at 375 F for 8 minutes.
6. Serve and enjoy.

438.Fennel And Parmesan Dip

Servings: 8
Cooking Time: 25 Minutes
Ingredients:
- 3 tablespoons olive oil
- 3 fennel bulbs, trimmed and cut into wedges
- A pinch of salt and black pepper
- 4 garlic cloves, minced
- ¼ cup parmesan, grated

Directions:
1. Put the fennel in the air fryer's basket and bake at 380 degrees F for 20 minutes. In a blender, combine the roasted fennel with the rest of the ingredients and pulse well. Put the spread in a ramekin, introduce it in the fryer and cook at 380 degrees F for 5 minutes more. Divide into bowls and serve as a dip.

439.Mozzarella, Brie And Artichoke Dip

Servings: 10
Cooking Time: 22 Minutes
Ingredients:
- 2 cups arugula leaves, torn into pieces
- 1/3 can artichoke hearts, drained and chopped
- 1/2 cup Mozzarella cheese, shredded
- 1/3 cup sour cream
- 3 cloves garlic, minced
- 1/3 teaspoon dried basil
- 1 teaspoon sea salt
- 7 ounces Brie cheese
- 1/2 cup mayonnaise
- 1/3 teaspoon ground black pepper, or more to taste
- A pinch of ground allspice

Directions:
1. Combine together the Brie cheese, mayonnaise, sour cream, garlic, basil, salt, ground black pepper, and the allspice.
2. Throw in the artichoke hearts and arugula; gently stir to combine. Transfer the prepared mixture to a baking dish. Now, scatter the Mozzarella cheese evenly over the top.
3. Bake in your Air Fryer at 325 degrees F for 17 minutes. Serve with keto veggie sticks. Bon appétit!

440.Healthy Vegetable Kabobs

Servings: 4
Cooking Time: 10 Minutes

Ingredients:
- 1/2 onion
- 1 zucchini
- 1 eggplant
- 2 bell peppers
- Pepper
- Salt

Directions:
1. Cut all vegetables into 1-inch pieces.
2. Thread vegetables onto the soaked wooden skewers and season with pepper and salt.
3. Place skewers into the air fryer basket and cook for 10 minutes at 390 F. Turn halfway through.
4. Serve and enjoy.

441.Vegetable Mix

Servings: 4
Cooking Time: 45 Minutes
Ingredients:
- 3.5 oz. radish
- ½ tsp. parsley
- 3.5 oz. celeriac
- 1 yellow carrot
- 1 orange carrot
- 1 red onion
- 3.5 oz. pumpkin
- 3.5 oz. parsnips
- Salt to taste
- Epaulette pepper to taste
- 1 tbsp. olive oil
- 4 cloves garlic, unpeeled

Directions:
1. Peel and slice up all the vegetables into 2- to 3-cm pieces.
2. Pre-heat your Air Fryer to 390°F.
3. Pour in the oil and allow it to warm before placing the vegetables in the fryer, followed by the garlic, salt and pepper.
4. Roast for 18 – 20 minutes.
5. Top with parsley and serve hot with rice if desired.

442.Romano Cheese And Broccoli Balls

Servings: 4
Cooking Time: 25 Minutes
Ingredients:
- 1/2 pound broccoli
- 1/2 cup Romano cheese, grated
- 2 garlic cloves, minced
- 1 shallot, chopped
- 4 eggs, beaten
- 2 tablespoons butter, at room temperature
- 1/2 teaspoon paprika
- 1/4 teaspoon dried basil
- Sea salt and ground black pepper, to taste

Directions:
1. Add the broccoli to your food processor and pulse until the consistency resembles rice.

2. Stir in the remaining ingredients; mix until everything is well combined. Shape the mixture into bite-sized balls and transfer them to the lightly greased cooking basket.
3. Cook in the preheated Air Fryer at 375 degrees F for 16 minutes, shaking halfway through the cooking time. Serve with cocktail sticks and tomato ketchup on the side.

443.Spinach Dip

Servings:8
Cooking Time: 40 Minutes
Ingredients:
- 8 oz cream cheese, softened
- 1/4 tsp garlic powder
- 1/2 cup onion, minced
- 1/3 cup water chestnuts, drained and chopped
- 1 cup mayonnaise
- 1 cup parmesan cheese, grated
- 1 cup frozen spinach, thawed and squeeze out all liquid
- 1/2 tsp pepper

Directions:
1. Spray air fryer baking dish with cooking spray.
2. Add all ingredients into the bowl and mix until well combined.
3. Transfer bowl mixture into the prepared baking dish and place dish in air fryer basket.
4. Cook at 300 F for 35-40 minutes. After 20 minutes of cooking stir dip.
5. Serve and enjoy.

444.Carrots & Cumin

Servings: 4
Cooking Time: 25 Minutes
Ingredients:
- 2 cups carrots, peeled and chopped
- 1 tsp. cumin seeds
- 1 tbsp. olive oil
- ¼ cup coriander

Directions:
1. Cover the carrots with the cumin and oil.
2. Transfer to the Air Fryer and cook at 390°F for 12 minutes.
3. Season with the coriander before serving.

445.Spicy Avocado Fries Wrapped In Bacon

Servings: 5
Cooking Time: 10 Minutes
Ingredients:
- 2 teaspoons chili powder
- 2 avocados, pitted and cut into 10 pieces
- 1 teaspoon salt
- ½ teaspoon garlic powder
- 1 teaspoon ground black pepper
- 5 rashers back bacon, cut into halves

Directions:
1. Lay the bacon rashers on a clean surface; then, place one piece of avocado slice on each bacon slice. Add the salt, black pepper, chili powder, and garlic powder.
2. Then, wrap the bacon slice around the avocado and repeat with the remaining rolls; secure them with a cocktail sticks or toothpicks.
3. Preheat your Air Fryer to 370 degrees F; cook in the preheated air fryer for 5 minutes and serve with your favorite sauce for dipping.

446.Bacon Asparagus Wraps

Servings: 8
Cooking Time: 15 Minutes
Ingredients:
- 16 asparagus spears, trimmed
- 16 bacon strips
- 2 tablespoons olive oil
- 1 tablespoon lemon juice
- 1 teaspoon thyme, chopped
- 1 teaspoon oregano, chopped
- A pinch of salt and black pepper

Directions:
1. In a bowl, mix the oil with lemon juice, the herbs, salt and pepper and whisk well. Brush the asparagus spears with this mix and wrap each in a bacon strip. Arrange the asparagus wraps in your air fryer's basket and cook at 390 degrees F for 15 minutes. Serve as an appetizer.

447.Zucchini Crackers

Servings:16
Cooking Time: 20 Minutes
Ingredients:
- 1 cup zucchini, grated
- 2 tablespoons flax meal
- 1 teaspoon salt
- 3 tablespoons almond flour
- ¼ teaspoon baking powder
- ¼ teaspoon chili flakes
- 1 tablespoon xanthan gum
- 1 tablespoon butter, softened
- 1 egg, beaten
- Cooking spray

Directions:
1. Squeeze the zucchini to get rid of vegetable juice and transfer in the big bowl. Add flax meal, salt, almond flour, baking powder, chili flakes, xanthan gum, and stir well. After this, add butter and egg. Knead the non-sticky dough. Place it on the baking paper and cover with the second sheet of baking paper. Roll up the dough into the flat square.

After this, remove the baking paper from the dough surface. Cut it on medium size crackers. Line the air fryer basket with baking paper and put the crackers inside in one layer. Spray them with cooking spray. Cook them at 355F for 20 minutes.

448.Curried Sweet Potato Fries

Servings: 3
Cooking Time: 20 Minutes
Ingredients:
- 2 small sweet potatoes, peel and cut into fries shape
- 1/4 tsp coriander
- 1/2 tsp curry powder
- 2 tbsp olive oil
- 1/4 tsp sea salt

Directions:
1. Add all ingredients into the large mixing bowl and toss well.
2. Spray air fryer basket with cooking spray.
3. Transfer sweet potato fries in the air fryer basket.
4. Cook for 20 minutes at 370 F. Shake halfway through.
5. Serve and enjoy.

449.Delightful Fish Nuggets

Servings:4
Cooking Time:10 Minutes
Ingredients:
- 1 cup all-purpose flour
- 2 eggs
- ¾ cup breadcrumbs
- 1 pound cod, cut into 1x2½-inch strips
- Pinch of salt
- 2 tablespoons olive oil

Directions:
1. Preheat the Air fryer to 380 °F and grease an Air fryer basket.
2. Place flour in a shallow dish and whisk the eggs in a second dish.
3. Mix breadcrumbs, salt and oil in a third shallow dish.
4. Coat the fish strips evenly in flour and dip in the egg.
5. Roll into the breadcrumbs evenly and arrange the nuggets in an Air fryer basket.
6. Cook for about 10 minutes and dish out to serve warm.

450.Veggie Sandwich

Servings:2
Cooking Time: 25 Minutes
Ingredients:
- For Barbecue Sauce:
- 1 teaspoon olive oil
- 1 garlic clove, minced
- ¼ of onion, chopped
- ½ cup water
- ½ tablespoon sugar
- ½ tablespoon Worcestershire sauce
- ¼ teaspoon mustard powder
- 1½ tablespoons tomato ketchup
- Salt and ground black pepper, as needed
- For Sandwich:
- 2 tablespoons butter, softened
- 1 cup sweet corn kernels
- 1 roasted green bell pepper, chopped
- 4 bread slices, trimmed and cut horizontally

Directions:
1. For barbecue sauce: in a medium skillet, heat the oil over medium heat and sauté the garlic, and onion for about 3-5 minutes.
2. Stir in the remaining ingredients and bring to a boil over high heat.
3. Reduce the heat to medium and simmer for about 8-10 minutes or until desired thickness.
4. For the sandwich: in a skillet, melt the butter on medium heat and stir fry the corn for about 1-2 minutes.
5. In a bowl, mix together the barbecue sauce, corn, and bell pepper.
6. Spread the corn mixture on one side of 2 bread slices.
7. Top with the remaining slices.
8. Set the temperature of Air Fryer to 355 degrees F.
9. Place the sandwiches in an Air Fryer basket in a single layer.
10. Air Fry for about 5-6 minutes.
11. Serve.

451.Paprika Potato Chips

Servings: 3
Cooking Time: 50 Minutes
Ingredients:
- 3 potatoes, thinly sliced
- 1 teaspoon sea salt
- 1 teaspoon garlic powder
- 1 teaspoon paprika
- 1/4 cup ketchup

Directions:
1. Add the sliced potatoes to a bowl with salted water. Let them soak for 30 minutes. Drain and rinse your potatoes.
2. Pat dry and toss with salt.
3. Cook in the preheated Air Fryer at 400 degrees F for 15 minutes, shaking the basket occasionally.
4. Work in batches. Toss with the garlic powder and paprika. Serve with ketchup. Enjoy!

452.Batter-fried Shallots

Servings: 4
Cooking Time: 25 Minutes

Ingredients:

- 1/2 cup almond flour
- 2 large-sized eggs
- 1/2 teaspoon baking powder
- 2/3 teaspoon red pepper flakes, crushed
- 1 cup shallots, sliced into rings
- 1/2 cup beer
- 1/2 teaspoon fine sea salt
- 1 cup pork rinds

Directions:

1. Start by preheating the Air Fryer for 7 to 10 minutes.
2. Then, use a medium-sized bowl to combine almond flour with eggs, baking powder, sea salt, beer and crushed red pepper flakes.
3. Dip shallots rings into the prepared batter; make sure to coat them on all sides. Now, coat them with the pork rinds.
4. Afterward, cook the shallots approximately 11 minutes at 345 degrees F. Eat warm.

453.Tuna Bowls

Servings: 2
Cooking Time: 10 Minutes
Ingredients:

- 1 pound tuna, skinless, boneless and cubed
- 3 scallion stalks, minced
- 1 chili pepper, minced
- 2 tablespoon olive oil
- 1 tablespoon coconut cream
- 1 tablespoon coconut aminos
- 2 tomatoes, cubed
- 1 teaspoon sesame seeds

Directions:

1. In a pan that fits your air fryer, mix all the ingredients except the sesame seeds, toss, introduce in the fryer and cook at 360 degrees F for 10 minutes. Divide into bowls and serve as an appetizer with sesame seeds sprinkled on top.

454.Chicken Stuffed Mushrooms

Servings:12
Cooking Time:15 Minutes
Ingredients:

- 12 large fresh mushrooms, stems removed
- 1 cup chicken meat, cubed
- ½ lb. imitation crabmeat, flaked
- 2 cups butter
- Garlic powder, to taste
- 2 cloves garlic, peeled and minced
- Salt and black pepper, to taste
- 1 (8 oz.) package cream cheese, softened
- Crushed red pepper, to taste

Directions:

1. Preheat the Air fryer to 375 °F and grease an Air fryer basket.
2. Heat butter on medium heat in a nonstick skillet and add chicken.

3. Sauté for about 5 minutes and stir in the remaining ingredients except mushrooms.
4. Stuff this filling mixture in the mushroom caps and arrange in the Air fryer basket.
5. Cook for about 10 minutes and dish out to serve warm.

455.Sesame Tortilla Chips

Servings:4
Cooking Time: 4 Minutes
Ingredients:

- 4 low carb tortillas
- ½ teaspoon salt
- 1 teaspoon sesame oil

Directions:

1. Cut the tortillas into the strips. Preheat the air fryer to 365F. Place the tortilla strips in the air fryer basket and sprinkle with sesame oil. Cook them for 3 minutes. Then give a shake to the chips and sprinkle with salt. Cook the chips for 1 minute more.

456.Cocktail Flanks

Servings: 4
Cooking Time: 45 Minutes
Ingredients:

- 1x 12-oz. package cocktail franks
- 1x 8-oz. can crescent rolls

Directions:

1. 1 Drain the cocktail franks and dry with paper towels.
2. 2 Unroll the crescent rolls and slice the dough into rectangular strips, roughly 1" by 1.5".
3. 3 Wrap the franks in the strips with the ends poking out. Leave in the freezer for 5 minutes.
4. 4 Pre-heat the Air Fryer to 330°F.
5. 5 Take the franks out of the freezer and put them in the cooking basket. Cook for 6 – 8 minutes.
6. 6 Reduce the heat to 390°F and cook for another 3 minutes or until a golden-brown color is achieved.

457.Cheese Filled Bell Peppers

Servings:3
Cooking Time:12 Minutes
Ingredients:

- 1 small green bell pepper
- 1 small red bell pepper
- 1 small yellow bell pepper
- ½ cup mozzarella cheese
- ½ cup cream cheese
- 3 teaspoons red chili flakes

Directions:

1. Preheat the Air fryer to 320 °F and grease an Air fryer basket.

2. Chop the tops of the bell peppers and remove all the seeds.
3. Mix together mozzarella cheese, cream cheese and red chili flakes in a bowl.
4. Stuff this cheese mixture in the bell peppers and put back the tops.
5. Arrange in the Air Fryer basket and cook for about 12 minutes.
6. Remove from the Air fryer and serve hot.

458.Beef Bites

Servings:2
Cooking Time: 15 Minutes
Ingredients:
- 1 teaspoon cayenne pepper
- 8 oz beef loin, chopped
- 1 tablespoon coconut flour
- 1 teaspoon nut oil
- ¼ teaspoon salt
- 1 teaspoon apple cider vinegar

Directions:
1. Sprinkle the beef with apple cider vinegar and salt. Then sprinkle it with cayenne pepper and coconut flour. Shake the meat well and transfer in the air fryer. Sprinkle it with nut oil and cook at 365F for 15 minutes. Shake the beef popcorn every 5 minutes to avoid burning.

459.Carrots & Rhubarb

Servings: 4
Cooking Time: 35 Minutes
Ingredients:
- 1 lb. heritage carrots
- 1 lb. rhubarb
- 1 medium orange
- ½ cup walnuts, halved
- 2 tsp. walnut oil
- ½ tsp. sugar or a few drops of sugar extract

Directions:
1. 1 Rinse the carrots to wash. Dry and chop them into 1-inch pieces.
2. 2 Transfer them to the Air Fryer basket and drizzle over the walnut oil.
3. 3 Cook at 320°F for about 20 minutes.
4. 4 In the meantime, wash the rhubarb and chop it into ½-inch pieces.
5. 5 Coarsely dice the walnuts.
6. 6 Wash the orange and grate its skin into a small bowl. Peel the rest of the orange and cut it up into wedges.
7. 7 Place the rhubarb, walnuts and sugar in the fryer and allow to cook for an additional 5 minutes.
8. 8 Add in 2 tbsp. of the orange zest, along with the orange wedges. Serve immediately.

460.Lemon Olives Dip

Servings: 6

Cooking Time: 5 Minutes
Ingredients:
- 1 cup black olives, pitted and chopped
- ¼ cup capers
- ½ cup olive oil
- 3 tablespoons lemon juice
- 2 garlic cloves, minced
- 2 teaspoon apple cider vinegar
- 1 cup parsley leaves
- 1 cup basil leaves
- A pinch of salt and black pepper

Directions:
1. In a blender, combine all the ingredients, pulse well and transfer to a ramekin. Place the ramekin in your air fryer's basket and cook at 350 degrees F for 5 minutes. Serve as a snack.

461.Parmesan Green Beans Sticks

Servings: 4
Cooking Time: 12 Minutes
Ingredients:
- 12 ounces green beans, trimmed
- 1 cup parmesan, grated
- 1 egg, whisked
- A pinch of salt and black pepper
- ¼ teaspoon sweet paprika

Directions:
1. In a bowl, mix the parmesan with salt, pepper and the paprika and stir. Put the egg in a separate bowl, Dredge the green beans in egg and then in the parmesan mix. Arrange the green beans in your air fryer's basket and cook at 380 degrees F for 12 minutes. Serve as a snack.

462.Garlic Potatoes

Servings: 4
Cooking Time: 40 Minutes
Ingredients:
- 1 lb. russet baking potatoes
- 1 tbsp. garlic powder
- 1 tbsp. freshly chopped parsley
- ½ tsp. salt
- ¼ tsp. black pepper
- 1 – 2 tbsp. olive oil

Directions:
1. Wash the potatoes and pat them dry with clean paper towels.
2. Pierce each potato several times with a fork.
3. Place the potatoes in a large bowl and season with the garlic powder, salt and pepper.
4. Pour over the olive oil and mix well.
5. Pre-heat the Air Fryer to 360°F.
6. Place the potatoes in the fryer and cook for about 30 minutes, shaking the basket a few times throughout the cooking time.

7. Garnish the potatoes with the chopped parsley and serve with butter, sour cream or another dipping sauce if desired.

463.Banana Peppers

Servings: 8
Cooking Time: 20 Minutes
Ingredients:
- 1 cup full-fat cream cheese
- Cooking spray
- 16 avocado slices
- 16 slices salami
- Salt and pepper to taste
- 16 banana peppers

Directions:
1. 1 Pre-heat the Air Fryer to 400°F.
2. 2 Spritz a baking tray with cooking spray.
3. 3 Remove the stems from the banana peppers with a knife.
4. 4 Cut a slit into one side of each banana pepper.
5. 5 Season the cream cheese with the salt and pepper and combine well.
6. 6 Fill each pepper with one spoonful of the cream cheese, followed by one slice of avocado.
7. 7 Wrap the banana peppers in the slices of salami and secure with a toothpick.
8. 8 Place the banana peppers in the baking tray and transfer it to the Air Fryer. Bake for roughly 8 - 10 minutes.

464.Roasted Cauliflower Florets

Servings: 2
Cooking Time: 20 Minutes
Ingredients:
- 3 cups cauliflower florets
- 2 teaspoons sesame oil
- 1 teaspoon onion powder
- 1 teaspoon garlic powder
- Sea salt and cracked black pepper, to taste
- 1 teaspoon paprika

Directions:
1. Start by preheating your Air Fryer to 400 degrees F.
2. Toss the cauliflower with the remaining ingredients; toss to coat well.
3. Cook for 12 minutes, shaking the cooking basket halfway through the cooking time. They will crisp up as they cool. Bon appétit!

465.Red Beet Chips With Pizza Sauce

Servings: 4
Cooking Time: 30 Minutes
Ingredients:
- 2 red beets, thinly sliced
- 1 tablespoon grapeseed oil
- 1 teaspoon seasoned salt
- 1/2 teaspoon ground black pepper

- 1/4 teaspoon cumin powder
- 1/2 cup pizza sauce

Directions:
1. Toss the red beets with the oil, salt, black pepper, and cumin powder.
2. Arrange the beet slices in a single layer in the Air Fryer basket.
3. Cook in the preheated Air Fryer at 330 degrees F for 13 minutes. Serve with the pizza sauce and enjoy!

466.Healthy Broccoli Tots

Servings: 4
Cooking Time: 25 Minutes
Ingredients:
- 1 lb broccoli, chopped
- 1/2 cup almond flour
- 1/4 cup ground flaxseed
- 1/2 tsp garlic powder
- 1 tsp salt

Directions:
1. Add broccoli into the microwave-safe bowl and microwave for 3 minutes.
2. Transfer steamed broccoli into the food processor and process until it looks like rice.
3. Transfer broccoli to a large mixing bowl.
4. Add remaining ingredients into the bowl and mix until well combined.
5. Spray air fryer basket with cooking spray.
6. Make small tots from broccoli mixture and place into the air fryer basket.
7. Cook broccoli tots for 12 minutes at 375 F.
8. Serve and enjoy.

467.Movie Night Zucchini Fries

Servings: 4
Cooking Time: 26 Minutes
Ingredients:
- 2 zucchinis, slice into sticks
- 2 teaspoons shallot powder
- 1/4 teaspoon dried dill weed
- 2 teaspoons garlic powder
- 1/2 cup Parmesan cheese, preferably freshly grated
- 1/3 teaspoon cayenne pepper
- 3 egg whites
- 1/3 cup almond meal
- Cooking spray
- Salt and ground black pepper, to your liking

Directions:
1. Pat the zucchini sticks dry using a kitchen towel.
2. Grab a mixing bowl and beat the egg whites until pale; then, add all the seasonings in the order listed above and beat again
3. Take another mixing bowl and mix together almond meal and the Parmesan cheese.

4. Then, coat the zucchini sticks with the seasoned egg mixture; then, roll them over the parmesan cheese mixture.
5. Lay the breaded zucchini sticks in a single layer on the tray that is coated lightly with cooking spray.
6. Bake at 375 degrees F for about 20 minutes until the sticks are golden brown. Serve with your favorite sauce for dipping.

468.Carrot Sticks

Servings:2
Cooking Time: 12 Minutes
Ingredients:
- 1 large carrot, peeled and cut into sticks
- 1 tablespoon fresh rosemary, finely chopped
- 1 tablespoon olive oil
- 2 teaspoons sugar
- ¼ teaspoon cayenne pepper
- Salt and freshly ground black pepper, as needed

Directions:
1. Set the temperature of Air Fryer to 390 degrees F.
2. In a bowl, add all the ingredients and toss to coat well.
3. Place the carrot sticks in an Air Fryer basket in a single layer.
4. Air Fry for about 12 minutes.
5. Serve.

469.Rangoon Crab Dip

Servings: 8
Cooking Time: 16 Minutes
Ingredients:
- 2 cups crab meat
- 1 cup mozzarella cheese, shredded
- 1/2 tsp garlic powder
- 1/4 cup pimentos, drained and diced
- 1/4 tsp stevia
- 1/2 lemon juice
- 2 tsp coconut amino
- 2 tsp mayonnaise
- 8 oz cream cheese, softened
- 1 tbsp green onion
- 1/4 tsp pepper
- Salt

Directions:
1. Preheat the air fryer to 325 F.
2. Add all ingredients except half mozzarella cheese into the large bowl and mix until well combined.
3. Transfer bowl mixture into the air fryer baking dish and sprinkle with remaining mozzarella cheese.
4. Place into the air fryer and cook for 16 minutes.
5. Serve and enjoy.

470.Cheesy Zucchini Sticks

Servings: 2
Cooking Time: 20 Minutes
Ingredients:
- 1 zucchini, slice into strips
- 2 tablespoons mayonnaise
- 1/4 cup tortilla chips, crushed
- 1/4 cup Romano cheese, shredded
- Sea salt and black pepper, to your liking
- 1 tablespoon garlic powder
- 1/2 teaspoon red pepper flakes

Directions:
1. Coat the zucchini with mayonnaise.
2. Mix the crushed tortilla chips, cheese and spices in a shallow dish.
3. Then, coat the zucchini sticks with the cheese/chips mixture.
4. Cook in the preheated Air Fryer at 400 degrees F for 12 minutes, shaking the basket halfway through the cooking time.
5. Work in batches until the sticks are crispy and golden brown. Bon appétit!

471.Crab Dip

Servings: 4
Cooking Time: 20 Minutes
Ingredients:
- 8 ounces cream cheese, soft
- 1 tablespoon lemon juice
- 1 cup coconut cream
- 1 tablespoon lemon juice
- 1 bunch green onions, minced
- 1 pound artichoke hearts, drained and chopped
- 12 ounces jumbo crab meat
- A pinch of salt and black pepper
- 1 and ½ cups mozzarella, shredded

Directions:
1. In a bowl, combine all the ingredients except half of the cheese and whisk them really well. Transfer this to a pan that fits your air fryer, introduce in the machine and cook at 400 degrees F for 15 minutes. Sprinkle the rest of the mozzarella on top and cook for 5 minutes more. Divide the mix into bowls and serve as a party dip.

472.Basic Salmon Croquettes

Servings:16
Cooking Time:14 Minutes
Ingredients:
- 1 large can red salmon, drained
- 2 eggs, lightly beaten
- 2 tablespoons fresh parsley, chopped
- 1 cup breadcrumbs
- 2 tablespoons milk
- Salt and black pepper, to taste
- 1/3 cup vegetable oil

Directions:
1. Preheat the Air fryer to 390 °F and grease an Air fryer basket.
2. Mash the salmon completely in a bowl and stir in eggs, parsley, breadcrumbs, milk, salt and black pepper.
3. Mix until well combined and make 16 equal-sized croquettes from the mixture.
4. Mix together oil and breadcrumbs in a shallow dish and coat the croquettes in this mixture.
5. Place half of the croquettes in the Air fryer basket and cook for about 7 minutes.
6. Repeat with the remaining croquettes and serve warm.

473.Bacon Fries

Servings: 2 – 4
Cooking Time: 60 Minutes
Ingredients:
- 2 large russet potatoes, peeled and cut into ½ inch sticks
- 5 slices of bacon, diced
- 2 tbsp. vegetable oil
- 2 ½ cups cheddar cheese, shredded
- 3 oz. cream cheese, melted
- Salt and freshly ground black pepper
- ¼ cup chopped scallions
- Ranch dressing

Directions:
1. 1 Boil a large pot of salted water.
2. 2 Briefly cook the potato sticks in the boiling water for 4 minutes.
3. 3 Drain the potatoes and run some cold water over them in order to wash off the starch. Pat them dry with a kitchen towel.
4. 4 Pre-heat the Air Fryer to 400°F.
5. 5 Put the chopped bacon in the Air Fryer and air-fry for 4 minutes. Shake the basket at the halfway point.
6. 6 Place the bacon on paper towels to drain any excess fat and remove the grease from the Air Fryer drawer.
7. 7 Coat the dried potatoes with oil and put them in the Air Fryer basket. Air-fry at 360°F for 25 minutes, giving the basket the occasional shake throughout the cooking time and sprinkling the fries with salt and freshly ground black pepper at the halfway point.
8. 8 Take a casserole dish or baking pan that is small enough to fit inside your Air Fryer and place the fries inside.
9. 9 Mix together the 2 cups of the Cheddar cheese and the melted cream cheese.
10. 10 Pour the cheese mixture over the fries and top them with the rest of the Cheddar cheese and the cooked bacon crumbles.
11. 11 Take absolute care when placing the baking pan inside the cooker. Use a foil sling

[a sheet of aluminum foil folded into a strip about 2 inches wide by 24 inches long].
12. 12 Cook the fries at 340°F for 5 minutes, ensuring the cheese melts.
13. 13 Garnish the fries with the chopped scallions and serve straight from in the baking dish with some ranch dressing.

474.Chocolate Cookie Dough Balls

Servings:6
Cooking Time: 20 Minutes
Ingredients:
- 16½ ounces store-bought chilled chocolate chip cookie dough
- ¼ cup butter, melted
- ½ cup chocolate cookie crumbs
- 2 tablespoons sugar

Directions:
1. Cut the cookie dough into 12 equal-sized pieces and then, shape each into a ball.
2. Add the melted butter in a shallow dish.
3. In another dish, mix together the cookie crumbs, and sugar.
4. Dip each cookie ball in the melted butter and then evenly coat with the cookie crumbs.
5. In the bottom of a baking sheet, place the coated cookie balls and freeze for at least 2 hours.
6. Preheat the air fryer to 350 degrees F.
7. Line the air fryer basket with a piece of foil.
8. Place the cookies balls in an Air Fryer basket in a single layer in 2 batches.
9. Air Fry for about 10 minutes.
10. Enjoy!

475.Salmon Croquettes

Servings:16
Cooking Time: 14 Minutes
Ingredients:
- 1 large can red salmon, drained
- 2 eggs, lightly beaten
- 2 tablespoons fresh parsley, chopped
- Salt and freshly ground black pepper, as needed
- 1/3 cup vegetable oil
- 1 cup breadcrumbs

Directions:
1. Set the temperature of Air Fryer to 390 degrees F.
2. In a bowl, add the salmon and mash it completely using a fork.
3. Add the eggs, parsley, salt, and black pepper. Mix until well combined.
4. Make 16 equal-sized croquettes from the mixture.
5. In a shallow dish, mix together the oil, and breadcrumbs.
6. Coat the croquettes evenly with the breadcrumb mixture.

7. Place the croquettes in an Air Fryer basket in a single layer in 2 batches.
8. Air Fry for about 7 minutes.
9. Serve.

476.Creamy Cheddar Eggs

Servings:8
Cooking Time: 16 Minutes
Ingredients:
- 4 eggs
- 2 oz pork rinds
- ¼ cup Cheddar cheese, shredded
- 1 tablespoon heavy cream
- 1 teaspoon fresh dill, chopped

Directions:
1. Place the eggs in the air fryer and cook them at 255F for 16 minutes. Then cool the eggs in the cold water and peel. Cut every egg into the halves and remove the egg yolks. Transfer the egg yolks in the mixing bowl. Add shredded cheese, heavy cream, and fresh dill. Stir the mixture with the help of the fork until smooth and add pork rinds. Mix it up. Fill the egg whites with the egg yolk mixture.

477.Mushroom Pizza Bites

Servings:6
Cooking Time: 7 Minutes
Ingredients:
- 6 cremini mushroom caps
- 3 oz Parmesan, grated
- 1 tablespoon olive oil
- ½ tomato, chopped
- ½ teaspoon dried basil
- 1 teaspoon ricotta cheese

Directions:
1. Preheat the air fryer to 400F. Sprinkle the mushroom caps with olive oil and put in the air fryer basket in one layer. Cook them for 3 minutes. After this, mix up tomato and ricotta cheese. Fill the mushroom caps with tomato mixture. Then top them with parmesan and sprinkle with dried basil. Cook the mushroom pizzas for 4 minutes at 400F.

478.Feta And Parsley Filo Triangles

Servings:6
Cooking Time:5 Minutes
Ingredients:
- 1 egg yolk
- 4-ounce feta cheese, crumbled
- 1 scallion, chopped finely
- 2 tablespoons fresh parsley, chopped finely
- 2 frozen filo pastry sheets, thawed and cut into three strips
- 2 tablespoons olive oil
- Salt and black pepper, to taste

Directions:
1. Preheat the Air fryer to 390 °F and grease an Air fryer basket.
2. Whisk egg yolk in a large bowl and beat well.
3. Stir in feta cheese, scallion, parsley, salt and black pepper.
4. Brush pastry with olive oil and put a tablespoon of feta mixture over one corner of filo strip.
5. Fold diagonally to create a triangle and keep folding until filling is completely wrapped.
6. Repeat with the remaining strips and filling and coat the triangles with olive oil.
7. Place the triangles in the Air fryer basket and cook for about 3 minutes.
8. Now, set the Air fryer to 360 degrees F and cook for another 2 minutes.
9. Dish out and serve warm.

479.Steak Nuggets

Servings: 4
Cooking Time: 15 Minutes
Ingredients:
- 1 lb beef steak, cut into chunks
- 1 large egg, lightly beaten
- 1/2 cup pork rind, crushed
- 1/2 cup parmesan cheese, grated
- 1/2 tsp salt

Directions:
1. Add egg in a small bowl.
2. In a shallow bowl, mix together pork rind, cheese, and salt.
3. Dip each steak chunk in egg then coat with pork rind mixture and place on a plate. Place in refrigerator for 30 minutes.
4. Spray air fryer basket with cooking spray.
5. Preheat the air fryer to 400 F.
6. Place steak nuggets in air fryer basket and cook for 15-18 minutes or until cooked. Shake after every 4 minutes.
7. Serve and enjoy.

480.Yakitori

Servings: 4
Cooking Time: 2 Hours 15 Minutes
Ingredients:
- 1/2 pound chicken tenders, cut bite-sized pieces
- 1 clove garlic, minced
- 1 teaspoon coriander seeds
- Sea salt and ground pepper, to taste
- 2 tablespoons Shoyu sauce
- 2 tablespoons sake
- 1 tablespoon fresh lemon juice
- 1 teaspoon sesame oil

Directions:
1. Place the chicken tenders, garlic, coriander, salt, black pepper, Shoyu sauce, sake, and

lemon juice in a ceramic dish; cover and let it marinate for 2 hours.

2. Then, discard the marinade and tread the chicken tenders onto bamboo skewers.
3. Place the skewered chicken in the lightly greased Air Fryer basket. Drizzle sesame oil all over the skewered chicken.
4. Cook at 360 degrees for 6 minutes. Turn the skewered chicken over; brush with the reserved marinade and cook for a further 6 minutes. Enjoy!

481.Rice Bites

Servings:4
Cooking Time: 20 Minutes
Ingredients:
- 3 cups cooked risotto
- 1/3 cup Parmesan cheese, grated
- 1 egg, beaten
- 3 ounces mozzarella cheese, cubed
- ¾ cup breadcrumbs

Directions:
1. In a bowl, mix together the risotto, Parmesan cheese, and egg.
2. Make 20 equal-sized balls from the mixture.
3. Insert a mozzarella cube in the center of each ball and using your fingers, smooth the risotto mixture to cover the mozzarella.
4. In a shallow dish, add the breadcrumbs.
5. Coat the balls evenly with breadcrumbs.
6. Set the temperature of Air Fryer to 390 degrees F.
7. Arrange the balls in an Air Fryer basket in a single layer in 2 batches.
8. Air Fry for about 10 minutes or until they turn golden brown.
9. Serve.

482.Bacon Wrapped Shrimp

Servings: 4
Cooking Time: 50 Minutes
Ingredients:
- 1 ¼ lb. tiger shrimp, peeled and deveined [16 pieces]
- 1 lb. bacon, thinly sliced, room temperature [16 slices]

Directions:
1. 1 Wrap each bacon slice around a piece of shrimp, from the head to the tail. Refrigerate for 20 minutes.
2. 2 Pre-heat the Air Fryer to 390°F.
3. 3 Place the shrimp in the fryer's basket and cook for 5 – 7 minutes.
4. 4 Allow to dry on a paper towel before serving.

483.Lemon Green Beans

Servings: 4
Cooking Time: 20 Minutes
Ingredients:

- 1 lemon, juiced
- 1 lb. green beans, washed and destemmed
- ¼ tsp. extra virgin olive oil
- Sea salt to taste
- Black pepper to taste

Directions:
1. Pre-heat the Air Fryer to 400°F.
2. Put the green beans in your Air Fryer basket and drizzle the lemon juice over them.
3. Sprinkle on the pepper and salt. Pour in the oil, and toss to coat the green beans well.
4. Cook for 10 – 12 minutes and serve warm.

484.Fried Kale Chips

Servings: 2
Cooking Time: 10 Minutes
Ingredients:
- 1 head kale, torn into 1 ½-inch pieces
- 1 tbsp. olive oil
- 1 tsp. soy sauce

Directions:
1. Wash and dry the kale pieces.
2. Transfer the kale to a bowl and coat with the soy sauce and oil.
3. Place it in the Air Fryer and cook at 400°F for 3 minutes, tossing it halfway through the cooking process.

485.Artichoke Dip

Servings: 6
Cooking Time: 24 Minutes
Ingredients:
- 15 oz artichoke hearts, drained
- 1 tsp Worcestershire sauce
- 3 cups arugula, chopped
- 1 cup cheddar cheese, shredded
- 1 tbsp onion, minced
- 1/2 cup mayonnaise

Directions:
1. Preheat the air fryer to 325 F.
2. Add all ingredients into the blender and blend until smooth.
3. Pour artichoke mixture into air fryer baking dish and place into the air fryer basket.
4. Cook dip for 24 minutes.
5. Serve with vegetables and enjoy.

486.Sweet Potato Bites

Servings: 2
Cooking Time: 30 Minutes
Ingredients:
- 2 sweet potatoes, diced into 1-inch cubes
- 1 tsp. red chili flakes
- 2 tsp. cinnamon
- 2 tbsp. olive oil
- 2 tbsp. honey
- ½ cup fresh parsley, chopped

Directions:
1. Pre-heat the Air Fryer at 350°F.

2. Place all of the ingredients in a bowl and stir well to coat the sweet potato cubes entirely.
3. Put the sweet potato mixture into the Air Fryer basket and cook for 15 minutes.

487.Cheese Boats

Servings: 2
Cooking Time: 30 Minutes
Ingredients:
- 1 cup ground chicken
- 1 zucchini
- 1 ½ cups crushed tomatoes
- ½ tsp. salt
- ¼ tsp. pepper
- ½ tsp. garlic powder
- 2 tbsp. butter or olive oil
- ½ cup cheese, grated
- ¼ tsp. dried oregano

Directions:
1. 1 Peel and halve the zucchini. Use a spoon to scoop out the flesh.
2. 2 In a bowl, combine the ground chicken, tomato, garlic powder, butter, cheese, oregano, salt, and pepper. Fill in the hollowed-out zucchini with this mixture.
3. 3 Transfer to the Air Fryer and bake for about 10 minutes at 400°F. Serve warm.

488.Feta Triangles

Servings: 5

Cooking Time: 55 Minutes
Ingredients:
- 1 egg yolk, beaten
- 4 oz. feta cheese
- 2 tbsp. flat-leafed parsley, finely chopped
- 1 scallion, finely chopped
- 2 sheets of frozen filo pastry, defrosted
- 2 tbsp. olive oil ground black pepper to taste

Directions:
1. 1 In a bowl, combine the beaten egg yolk with the feta, parsley and scallion. Sprinkle on some pepper to taste.
2. 2 Slice each sheet of filo dough into three strips.
3. 3 Place a teaspoonful of the feta mixture on each strip of pastry.
4. 4 Pinch the tip of the pastry and fold it up to enclose the filling and create a triangle. Continue folding the strip in zig-zags until the filling is wrapped in a triangle. Repeat with all of the strips of pastry.
5. 5 Pre-heat the Air Fryer to 390°F.
6. 6 Coat the pastry with a light coating of oil and arrange in the cooking basket.
7. 7 Place the basket in the Air Fryer and cook for 3 minutes.
8. 8 Lower the heat to 360°F and cook for a further 2 minutes or until a golden brown color is achieved

DESSERTS RECIPES

489.Chocolate Coconut Cake

Servings: 9
Cooking Time: 20 Minutes
Ingredients:
- 6 eggs
- 2 tsp baking powder
- 3 oz unsweetened cocoa powder
- 5 oz erythritol
- 3.5 oz coconut flour
- 1 tsp vanilla
- 3 oz butter, melted
- 11 oz heavy cream

Directions:
1. Preheat the air fryer to 325 F.
2. In a bowl, mix together coconut flour, butter, 5 oz heavy cream, eggs, baking powder half cocoa powder, and 3 oz sweetener until well combined.
3. Pour batter into the greased cake pan and place into the air fryer and cook for 20 minutes.
4. Allow to cool completely.
5. In a large bowl, beat remaining heavy cream, cocoa powder, and sweetener until smooth.
6. Spread the cream on top of cake and place in the refrigerator for 30 minutes.
7. Slice and serve.

490.Perfect Mini Cheesecakes

Servings: 6
Cooking Time: 40 Minutes + Chilling Time
Ingredients:
- 1/2 cup almond flour
- 1 ½ tablespoons unsalted butter, melted
- 2 tablespoons erythritol
- 1 (8-ounce) package cream cheese, softened
- 1/4 cup powdered erythritol
- 1/2 teaspoon vanilla paste
- 1 egg, at room temperature
- Topping:
- 1 ½ cups sour cream
- 3 tablespoons powdered erythritol
- 1 teaspoon vanilla extract

Directions:
1. Thoroughly combine the almond flour, butter, and 2 tablespoons of erythritol in a mixing bowl. Press the mixture into the bottom of lightly greased custard cups.
2. Then, mix the cream cheese, 1/4 cup of powdered erythritol, vanilla, and egg using an electric mixer on low speed. Pour the batter into the pan, covering the crust.
3. Bake in the preheated Air Fryer at 330 degrees F for 35 minutes until edges are puffed and the surface is firm.
4. Mix the sour cream, 3 tablespoons of powdered erythritol, and vanilla for the topping; spread over the crust and allow it to cool to room temperature.
5. Transfer to your refrigerator for 6 to 8 hours. Serve well chilled.

491.White Chocolate Rum Molten Cake

Servings: 4
Cooking Time: 20 Minutes
Ingredients:
- 2 ½ ounces butter, at room temperature
- 3 ounces white chocolate
- 2 eggs, beaten
- 1/2 cup powdered sugar
- 1/3 cup self-rising flour
- 1 teaspoon rum extract
- 1 teaspoon vanilla extract

Directions:
1. Begin by preheating your Air Fryer to 370 degrees F. Spritz the sides and bottom of four ramekins with cooking spray.
2. Melt the butter and white chocolate in a microwave-safe bowl. Mix the eggs and sugar until frothy.
3. Pour the butter/chocolate mixture into the egg mixture. Stir in the flour, rum extract, and vanilla extract. Mix until everything is well incorporated.
4. Scrape the batter into the prepared ramekins. Bake in the preheated Air Fryer for 9 to 11 minutes.
5. Let stand for 2 to 3 minutes. Invert on a plate while warm and serve. Bon appétt!

492.Sponge Cake

Servings: 8
Cooking Time: 50 Minutes
Ingredients:
- For the Cake:
- 9 oz. sugar
- 9 oz. butter
- 3 eggs
- 9 oz. flour
- 1 tsp. vanilla extract
- Zest of 1 lemon
- 1 tsp. baking powder
- For the Frosting
- Juice of 1 lemon
- Zest of 1 lemon
- 1 tsp. yellow food coloring
- 7 oz. sugar
- 4 egg whites

Directions:
1. Pre-heat your Air Fryer to 320°F.
2. Use an electric mixer to combine all of the cake ingredients.

3. Grease the insides of two round cake pans.
4. Pour an equal amount of the batter into each pan.
5. Place one pan in the fryer and cook for 15 minutes, before repeating with the second pan.
6. In the meantime, mix together all of the frosting ingredients.
7. Allow the cakes to cool. Spread the frosting on top of one cake and stack the other cake on top.

493.Nut Bars

Servings: 10
Cooking Time: 30 Minutes
Ingredients:
- ½ cup coconut oil, softened
- 1 teaspoon baking powder
- 1 teaspoon lemon juice
- 1 cup almond flour
- ½ cup coconut flour
- 3 tablespoons Erythritol
- 1 teaspoon vanilla extract
- 2 eggs, beaten
- 2 oz hazelnuts, chopped
- 1 oz macadamia nuts, chopped
- Cooking spray

Directions:
1. In the mixing bowl mix up coconut oil and baking powder. Add lemon juice, almond flour, coconut flour, Erythritol, vanilla extract, and eggs. Stir the mixture until it is smooth or use the immersion blender for this step. Then add hazelnuts and macadamia nuts. Stir the mixture until homogenous. After this, preheat the air fryer to 325F. Line the air fryer basket with baking paper. Then pour the nut mixture in the air fryer basket and flatten it well with the help of the spatula. Cook the mixture for 30 minutes. Then cool the mixture well and cut it into the serving bars.

494.Coffee 'n Blueberry Cake

Servings:6
Cooking Time: 35 Minutes
Ingredients:
- 1 cup white sugar
- 1 egg
- 1/2 cup butter, softened
- 1/2 cup fresh or frozen blueberries
- 1/2 cup sour cream
- 1/2 teaspoon baking powder
- 1/2 teaspoon ground cinnamon
- 1/2 teaspoon vanilla extract
- 1/4 cup brown sugar
- 1/4 cup chopped pecans
- 1/8 teaspoon salt

- 1-1/2 teaspoons confectioners' sugar for dusting
- 3/4 cup and 1 tablespoon all-purpose flour

Directions:
1. In a small bowl, whisk well pecans, cinnamon, and brown sugar.
2. In a blender, blend well all wet Ingredients. Add dry Ingredients except for confectioner's sugar and blueberries. Blend well until smooth and creamy.
3. Lightly grease baking pan of air fryer with cooking spray.
4. Pour half of batter in pan. Sprinkle half of pecan mixture on top. Pour the remaining batter. And then topped with remaining pecan mixture.
5. Cover pan with foil.
6. For 35 minutes, cook on 330 °F.
7. Serve and enjoy with a dusting of confectioner's sugar.

495.Cashew Bars Recipe

Servings: 6
Cooking Time:25 Minutes
Ingredients:
- 1/4 cup almond meal
- 1 tbsp. almond butter
- 1 ½ cups cashews; chopped
- 4 dates; chopped
- 3/4 cup coconut; shredded
- 1/3 cup honey
- 1 tbsp. chia seeds

Directions:
1. In a bowl; mix honey with almond meal and almond butter and stir well.
2. Add cashews, coconut, dates and chia seeds and stir well again.
3. Spread this on a lined baking sheet that fits your air fryer and press well.
4. Introduce in the fryer and cook at 300 °F, for 15 minutes. Leave mix to cool down, cut into medium bars and serve

496.Mini Apple Pies

Servings:6
Cooking Time: 30 Minutes
Ingredients:
- For Crust:
- 1½ cups flour
- 1 teaspoon sugar
- Salt, to taste
- ½ cup unsalted butter
- ¼ cup chilled water
- For Filling:
- 4 Granny Smith apples, peeled and finely chopped
- 1 teaspoon fresh lemon zest, finely grated
- 2½ tablespoons sugar
- 2 tablespoons flour

- 1 teaspoon ground cinnamon
- ¼ teaspoon ground nutmeg
- Salt, to taste
- ¼ cup Nutella
- 2 tablespoons fresh lemon juice
- 2 tablespoons butter
- For Topping:
- 1 egg, beaten
- 3 tablespoons sugar
- 1 teaspoon ground cinnamon

Directions:
1. In a bowl, mix well flour, sugar, butter, and salt.
2. With a pastry cutter, cut in the butter.
3. Add the chilled water and mix until a dough forms.
4. With a plastic wrapper, cover the bowl and refrigerate for about 30 minutes.
5. Meanwhile, for filling: in a large bowl, mix well all the ingredients. Set aside.
6. Now, place the dough onto a lightly floured surface and roll into ½-inch thickness.
7. With a ramekin, cut 12 circles from the dough.
8. Place 6 circles in the bottom of 6 ramekins and press slightly.
9. Add the filling mixture evenly into the ramekins and top with the remaining circles.
10. Pinch the edges to seal the pies.
11. Carefully, cut 3 slits in each pie and coat evenly with the beaten egg.
12. For topping: in a small bowl, mix together the cinnamon and sugar.
13. Sprinkle each pie with the cinnamon sugar.
14. Set the temperature of air fryer to 350 degrees F.
15. Arrange the ramekins into an air fryer basket.
16. Air fry for about 30 minutes.
17. Remove the ramekins from air fryer and place onto a wire rack to cool for about 10-15 minutes before serving.
18. Serve warm.

497.Blackberry And Cocoa Butter Cake

Servings: 8
Cooking Time: 30 Minutes
Ingredients:
- 1/3 cup fresh blackberries
- 1/2 cup butter, room temperature
- 1/3 teaspoon baking powder
- 2 ounces swerve
- 1/2 cup cocoa powder, melted
- 1 teaspoon baking soda
- 4 whole eggs
- 1 cup almond flour
- 1 teaspoon orange zest

Directions:

1. In a bowl, beat the butter, swerve and orange zest with an electric mixer. Carefully fold in the eggs, one at a time; beat well with your electric mixer after each addition.
2. Next, throw in the almond flour, baking soda, baking powder, cocoa powder, and orange juice.
3. Pour the prepared batter into a loaf pan. Top with fresh blackberries. Bake in the preheated Air Fryer for 22 minutes at 335 degrees F.
4. Check the cake for doneness; allow it to cool on a wire rack. Bon appétit!

498.Cinnamon And Butter Pancakes

Servings: 2
Cooking Time: 12 Minutes
Ingredients:
- 1 teaspoon ground cinnamon
- 2 teaspoons butter, softened
- 1 teaspoon baking powder
- ½ teaspoon lemon juice
- ½ teaspoon vanilla extract
- ¼ cup heavy cream
- 4 tablespoons almond flour
- 2 teaspoons Erythritol

Directions:
1. Preheat the air fryer to 325F. Take 2 small cake mold and line them with baking paper. After this, in the mixing bowl mix up ground cinnamon, butter, baking powder, lemon juice, vanilla extract, heavy cream, almond flour, and Erythritol. Stir the mixture until it is smooth. Then pour the mixture in the prepared cake molds. Put the first cake mold in the air fryer and cook the pancake for 6 minutes. Then check if the pancake is cooked (it should have light brown color) and remove it from the air fryer. Repeat the same steps with the second pancake. It is recommended to serve the pancakes warm or hot.

499.Sweet Coconut Cream Pie

Servings: 4
Cooking Time: 25 Minutes
Ingredients:
- 4 tablespoons coconut cream
- 1 teaspoon baking powder
- 1 teaspoon apple cider vinegar
- 1 egg, beaten
- ¼ cup coconut flakes
- 1 teaspoon vanilla extract
- ½ cup coconut flour
- 4 teaspoons Splenda
- 1 teaspoon xanthan gum
- Cooking spray

Directions:

1. Put all liquid ingredients in the bowl: coconut cream, apple cider vinegar, egg, and vanilla extract. Stir the liquid until homogenous and add baking powder, coconut flakes, coconut flour, Splenda, and xanthan gum. Stir the ingredients until you get the smooth texture of the batter. Spray the air fryer cake mold with cooking spray. Pour the batter in the cake mold. Preheat the air fryer to 330F. Put the cake mold in the air fryer basket and cook it for 25 minutes. Then cool the cooked pie completely and remove it from the cake mold. Cut the cooked pie into servings.

500.Marshmallow Pastries

Servings:8
Cooking Time:5 Minutes
Ingredients:
- 4-ounce butter, melted
- 8 phyllo pastry sheets, thawed
- ½ cup chunky peanut butter
- 8 teaspoons marshmallow fluff
- Pinch of salt

Directions:
1. Preheat the Air fryer to 360 °F and grease an Air fryer basket.
2. Brush butter over 1 filo pastry sheet and top with a second filo sheet.
3. Brush butter over second filo pastry sheet and repeat with all the remaining sheets.
4. Cut the phyllo layers in 8 strips and put 1 tablespoon of peanut butter and 1 teaspoon of marshmallow fluff on the underside of a filo strip.
5. Fold the tip of the sheet over the filling to form a triangle and fold repeatedly in a zigzag manner.
6. Arrange the pastries into the Air fryer basket and cook for about 5 minutes.
7. Season with a pinch of salt and serve warm.

501.Coconut And Berries Cream

Servings: 6
Cooking Time: 30 Minutes
Ingredients:
- 12 ounces blackberries
- 6 ounces raspberries
- 12 ounces blueberries
- ¾ cup swerve
- 2 ounces coconut cream

Directions:
1. In a bowl, mix all the ingredients and whisk well. Divide this into 6 ramekins, put them in your air fryer and cook at 320 degrees F for 30 minutes. Cool down and serve it.

502.Coconut Pillow

Servings: 4

Cooking Time: 1-2 Days
Ingredients:
- 1 can unsweetened coconut milk
- Berries of choice
- Dark chocolate

Directions:
1. Refrigerate the coconut milk for 24 hours.
2. Remove it from your refrigerator and whip for 2-3 minutes.
3. Fold in the berries.
4. Season with the chocolate shavings.
5. Serve!

503.Cinnamon Donuts

Servings: 4
Cooking Time: 6 Minutes
Ingredients:
- 1 teaspoon ground cardamom
- ½ teaspoon ground cinnamon
- ½ teaspoon baking powder
- ½ cup coconut flour
- 1 tablespoon Erythritol
- 1 egg, beaten
- 1 tablespoon butter, softened
- ¼ teaspoon salt
- Cooking spray

Directions:
1. Preheat the air fryer to 355F. In the shallow bowl mix up ground cinnamon, ground cardamom, and Erythritol. After this, in the separated bowl mix up coconut flour, baking powder, egg, salt, and butter. Knead the non-sticky dough. Add more coconut flour if needed. Then roll up the dough and make 4 donuts with the help of the donut cutter. After this, coat every donut in the cardamom mixture. Let the donuts rest for 10 minutes in a warm place. Then spray the air fryer with cooking spray. Place the donuts in the air fryer basket in one layer and cook them for 6 minutes or until they are golden brown. Sprinkle the hot cooked donuts with the remaining cardamom mixture.

504.Pop Tarts With Homemade Strawberry Jam

Servings: 8
Cooking Time: 45 Minutes
Ingredients:
- 1 cup strawberries, sliced
- 1 tablespoon fresh lemon juice
- 1 teaspoon maple syrup
- 2 tablespoons chia seeds
- 1 (14-ounce) box refrigerated pie crust
- 1 egg, whisked with 1 tablespoon of water (egg wash)
- 1/2 cup powdered sugar

Directions:

1. In a saucepan, heat the strawberries until they start to get syrupy. Mash them and add the lemon juice and maple syrup.
2. Remove from the heat and stir in the chia seeds. Let it stand for 30 minutes or until it thickens up.
3. Unroll the pie crusts and cut them into small rectangles. Spoon the strawberry jam in the center of a rectangle; top with another piece of crust.
4. Repeat until you run out of ingredients. Line the Air Fryer basket with parchment paper.
5. Brush the pop tarts with the egg wash and bake at 400 degrees F for 6 minutes or until slightly brown. Work in batches and transfer to cooling racks.
6. Dust with powdered sugar and enjoy!

505.Creamy Nutmeg Cake

Servings: 8
Cooking Time: 40 Minutes
Ingredients:
- ½ cup heavy cream
- 3 eggs, beaten
- 3 tablespoons cocoa powder
- 1 teaspoon vanilla extract
- 1 teaspoon baking powder
- 3 tablespoons Erythritol
- 1 cup almond flour
- ¼ teaspoon ground nutmeg
- 1 tablespoon avocado oil
- 1 teaspoon Splenda

Directions:
1. Mix up heavy cream and eggs in the bowl. Add cocoa powder and stir the liquid until it is smooth. After this, add vanilla extract, baking powder, Erythritol, almond flour, ground nutmeg, and avocado oil. Whisk the mixture gently and pour it in the cake mold. Then cover the cake with foil. Secure the edges of the foil. Then pierce the foil with the help of the toothpick. Preheat the air fryer to 360F. Put the cake mold in the air fryer and cook it for 40 minutes. When the cake is cooked, remove it from the air fryer and cool completely. Remove the cake from the mold and them sprinkle with Splenda.

506.Yummy Banana Cookies

Servings:6
Cooking Time: 10 Minutes
Ingredients:
- 1 cup dates, pitted and chopped
- 1 teaspoon vanilla
- 1/3 cup vegetable oil
- 2 cups rolled oats
- 3 ripe bananas

Directions:
1. Preheat the air fryer to 350°F.

2. In a bowl, mash the bananas and add in the rest of the ingredients.
3. Let it rest inside the fridge for 10 minutes.
4. Drop a teaspoonful on cut parchment paper.
5. Place the cookies on parchment paper inside the air fryer basket. Make sure that the cookies do not overlap.
6. Cook for 20 minutes or until the edges are crispy.
7. Serve with almond milk.

507.Easy Baked Chocolate Mug Cake

Servings:3
Cooking Time: 15 Minutes
Ingredients:
- ½ cup cocoa powder
- ½ cup stevia powder
- 1 cup coconut cream
- 1 package cream cheese, room temperature
- 1 tablespoon vanilla extract
- 4 tablespoons butter

Directions:
1. Preheat the air fryer for 5 minutes.
2. In a mixing bowl, combine all ingredients.
3. Use a hand mixer to mix everything until fluffy.
4. Pour into greased mugs.
5. Place the mugs in the fryer basket.
6. Bake for 15 minutes at 350°F.
7. Place in the fridge to chill before serving.

508.Orange Carrot Cake

Servings: 8
Cooking Time: 30 Minutes
Ingredients:
- 2 large carrots, peeled and grated
- 1 ¾ cup flour
- ¾ cup sugar
- 2 eggs
- 10 tbsp. olive oil
- 2 cups sugar
- 1 tsp. mixed spice
- 2 tbsp. milk
- 4 tbsp. melted butter
- 1 small orange, rind and juice

Directions:
1. Set the Air Fryer to 360°F and allow to heat up for 10 minutes.
2. Place a baking sheet inside the tin.
3. Combine the flour, sugar, grated carrots, and mixed spice.
4. Pour the milk, beaten eggs, and olive oil into the middle of the batter and mix well.
5. Pour the mixture in the tin, transfer to the fryer and cook for 5 minutes.
6. Lower the heat to 320°F and allow to cook for an additional 5 minutes.
7. In the meantime, prepare the frosting by combining the melted butter, orange juice,

rind, and sugar until a smooth consistency is achieved.
8. Remove the cake from the fryer, allow it to cool for several minutes and add the frosting on top.

509.English Lemon Tarts

Servings: 4
Cooking Time: 30 Minutes
Ingredients:
- ½ cup butter
- ½ lb. flour
- 2 tbsp. sugar
- 1 large lemon, juiced and zested
- 2 tbsp. lemon curd
- Pinch of nutmeg

Directions:
1. In a large bowl, combine the butter, flour and sugar until a crumbly consistency is achieved.
2. Add in the lemon zest and juice, followed by a pinch of nutmeg. Continue to combine. If necessary, add a couple tablespoons of water to soften the dough.
3. Sprinkle the insides of a few small pastry tins with flour. Pour equal portions of the dough into each one and add sugar or lemon zest on top.
4. Pre-heat the Air Fryer to 360°F.
5. Place the lemon tarts inside the fryer and allow to cook for 15 minutes.

510.Aromatic Cup

Servings: 1
Cooking Time: 15 Minutes
Ingredients:
- 1 egg, beaten
- 1 tablespoon peanut butter
- ½ teaspoon baking powder
- 1 teaspoon lemon juice
- ½ teaspoon vanilla extract
- 1 teaspoon Erythritol
- 2 tablespoons coconut flour

Directions:
1. Mix up all ingredients in the cup until homogenous. Then preheat the air fryer to 350F. Put the cup with blondies in the air fryer and cook it for 15 minutes.

511.Plum Bars Recipe

Servings: 8
Cooking Time:26 Minutes
Ingredients:
- 2 cups dried plums
- 6 tbsp. water
- 2 tbsp. butter; melted
- 1 egg; whisked
- 2 cup rolled oats
- 1 cup brown sugar

- ½ tsp. baking soda
- 1 tsp. cinnamon powder
- Cooking spray

Directions:
1. In your food processor, mix plums with water and blend until you obtain a sticky spread.
2. In a bowl; mix oats with cinnamon, baking soda, sugar, egg and butter and whisk really well.
3. Press half of the oats mix in a baking pan that fits your air fryer sprayed with cooking oil, spread plums mix and top with the other half of the oats mix
4. Introduce in your air fryer and cook at 350 °F, for 16 minutes. Leave mix aside to cool down, cut into medium bars and serve

512.Chia Cinnamon Pudding

Servings: 6
Cooking Time: 25 Minutes
Ingredients:
- 2 cups coconut cream
- 6 egg yolks, whisked
- 2 tablespoons stevia
- ¼ cup chia seeds
- 2 teaspoons cinnamon powder
- 1 tablespoon ghee, melted

Directions:
1. In a bowl, mix all the ingredients, whisk, divide into 6 ramekins, place them all in your air fryer and cook at 340 degrees F for 25 minutes. Cool the puddings down and serve.

513.Fruity Tacos

Servings:2
Cooking Time: 5 Minutes
Ingredients:
- 2 soft shell tortillas
- 4 tablespoons strawberry jelly
- ¼ cup blueberries
- ¼ cup raspberries
- 2 tablespoons powdered sugar

Directions:
1. Set the temperature of air fryer to 300 degrees F. Lightly, grease an air fryer basket.
2. Arrange the tortillas onto a smooth surface.
3. Spread two tablespoons of strawberry jelly over each tortilla and top each with berries.
4. Sprinkle each with the powdered sugar.
5. Arrange tortillas into the prepared air fryer basket.
6. Air fry for about 5 minutes or until crispy.
7. Remove from the air fryer and transfer the tortillas onto a platter.
8. Serve warm.

514.The Ultimate Berry Crumble

Servings: 6
Cooking Time: 40 Minutes
Ingredients:
- 18 ounces cherries
- 1/2 cup granulated sugar
- 2 tablespoons cornmeal
- 1/4 teaspoon ground star anise
- 1/2 teaspoon ground cinnamon
- 2/3 cup all-purpose flour
- 1 cup demerara sugar
- 1/2 teaspoon baking powder
- 1/3 cup rolled oats
- 1/2 stick butter, cut into small pieces

Directions:
1. Toss the cherries with the granulated sugar, cornmeal, star anise, and cinnamon. Divide between six custard cups coated with cooking spray.
2. In a mixing dish, thoroughly combine the remaining ingredients. Sprinkle over the berry mixture.
3. Bake in the preheated Air Fryer at 330 degrees F for 35 minutes. Bon appétit!

515.Apple Bread Pudding

Servings:8
Cooking Time: 44 Minutes
Ingredients:
- For Bread Pudding:
- 10½ ounces bread, cubed
- ½ cup apple, peeled, cored and chopped
- ½ cup raisins
- ¼ cup walnuts, chopped
- 1½ cups milk
- ¾ cup water
- 5 tablespoons honey
- 2 teaspoons ground cinnamon
- 2 teaspoons cornstarch
- 1 teaspoon vanilla extract
- For Topping:
- 1 1/3 cups plain flour
- 3/5 cup brown sugar
- 7 tablespoons butter

Directions:
1. In a large bowl, mix well bread, apple, raisins, and walnuts.
2. In another bowl, add the remaining pudding ingredients and mix until well combined.
3. Add the milk mixture into bread mixture and mix until well combined.
4. Refrigerate for about 15 minutes, tossing occasionally.
5. For topping: in a bowl, mix together the flour and sugar.
6. With a pastry cutter, cut in the butter until a crumbly mixture forms.

7. Set the temperature of air fryer to 355 degrees F.
8. Place the mixture evenly into 2 baking pans and spread the topping mixture on top of each.
9. Place 1 pan into an air fryer basket.
10. Air fry for about 22 minutes.
11. Repeat with the remaining pan.
12. Remove from the air fryer and serve warm.

516.Lemon Coconut Bars

Servings: 12
Cooking Time: 20 Minutes
Ingredients:
- 1 cup coconut cream
- ¼ cup cashew butter, soft
- ¾ cup swerve
- 1 egg, whisked
- Juice of 1 lemon
- 1 teaspoon lemon peel, grated
- 1 teaspoon baking powder

Directions:
1. In a bowl, combine all the ingredients gradually and stir well. Spoon balls this on a baking sheet lined with parchment paper and flatten them. Put the sheet in the fryer and cook at 350 degrees F for 20 minutes. Cut into bars and serve cold.

517.Chia Pudding

Servings: 1
Cooking Time: 10 Minutes
Ingredients:
- cup chia seeds
- 1 cup unsweetened coconut milk
- 1 tsp. liquid Sugar
- 1 tbsp. coconut oil
- 1 tsp. butter

Directions:
1. Pre-heat the fryer at 360°F.
2. In a bowl, gently combine the chia seeds with the milk and Sugar, before mixing the coconut oil and butter. Spoon seven equal-sized portions into seven ramekins and set these inside the fryer.
3. Cook for four minutes. Take care when removing the ramekins from the fryer and allow to cool for four minutes before serving.

518.Baked Peaches With Oatmeal Pecan Streusel

Servings: 3
Cooking Time: 20 Minutes
Ingredients:
- 2 tablespoons old-fashioned rolled oats
- 3 tablespoons golden caster sugar
- 1/2 teaspoon ground cinnamon
- 1 egg

- 2 tablespoons cold salted butter, cut into pieces
- 3 tablespoons pecans, chopped
- 3 large ripe freestone peaches, halved and pitted

Directions:
1. Mix the rolled oats, sugar, cinnamon, egg, and butter until well combined.
2. Add a big spoonful of prepared topping to the center of each peach. Pour 1/2 cup of water into an Air Fryer safe dish. Place the peaches in the dish.
3. Top the peaches with the roughly chopped pecans. Bake at 340 degrees F for 17 minutes. Serve at room temperature. Bon appétit!

519.Semolina Cake

Servings:8
Cooking Time:15 Minutes
Ingredients:
- 2½ cups semolina
- 1 cup milk
- 1 cup Greek yogurt
- 2 teaspoons baking powder
- ½ cup walnuts, chopped
- ½ cup vegetable oil
- 1 cup sugar
- Pinch of salt

Directions:
1. Preheat the Air fryer to 360 °F and grease a baking pan lightly.
2. Mix semolina, oil, milk, yogurt and sugar in a bowl until well combined.
3. Cover the bowl and keep aside for about 15 minutes.
4. Stir in the baking soda, baking powder and salt and fold in the walnuts.
5. Transfer the mixture into the baking pan and place in the Air fryer.
6. Cook for about 15 minutes and dish out to serve.

520.Sesame Bars

Servings: 6
Cooking Time: 10 Minutes
Ingredients:
- 1 cup coconut flour
- 2 tablespoons coconut flakes
- 2 eggs, beaten
- 1 teaspoon baking powder
- ¼ cup Erythritol
- 1 teaspoon vanilla extract
- 1 tablespoon butter, softened
- 1 teaspoon sesame seeds
- Cooking spray

Directions:
1. Put coconut flour in the bowl. Add coconut flakes, eggs, baking powder, Erythritol,

vanilla extract, and sesame seeds. Add butter. Stir the mixture with the help of the spoon until it is homogenous. Then roll up the dough into the square and cut into the bars. Preheat the air fryer to 325F, Line the air fryer with baking paper and put the coconut bars inside. Cook the coconut bars for 10 minutes.

521.Espresso Brownies With Mascarpone Frosting

Servings: 8
Cooking Time: 40 Minutes
Ingredients:
- 5 ounces unsweetened chocolate, chopped into chunks
- 2 tablespoons instant espresso powder
- 1 tablespoon cocoa powder, unsweetened
- 1/2 cup almond butter
- 1/2 cup almond meal
- 3/4 cup swerve
- 1 teaspoon pure coffee extract
- 1/2 teaspoon lime peel zest
- 1/4 cup coconut flour
- 2 eggs plus 1 egg yolk
- 1/2 teaspoon baking soda
- 1/2 teaspoon baking powder
- 1/2 teaspoon ground cinnamon
- 1/3 teaspoon ancho chile powder
- For the Chocolate Mascarpone Frosting:
- 4 ounces mascarpone cheese, at room temperature
- 1 ½ ounces unsweetened chocolate chips
- 1 ½ cups confectioner's swerve
- 1/4 cup unsalted butter, at room temperature
- 1 teaspoon vanilla paste
- A pinch of fine sea salt

Directions:
1. First of all, microwave the chocolate and almond butter until completely melted; allow the mixture to cool at room temperature.
2. Then, whisk the eggs, swerve, cinnamon, espresso powder, coffee extract, ancho chile powder, and lime zest.
3. Next step, add the vanilla/egg mixture to the chocolate/butter mixture. Stir in the almond meal and coconut flour along with baking soda, baking powder and cocoa powder.
4. Finally, press the batter into a lightly buttered cake pan. Air-fry for 35 minutes at 345 degrees F.
5. In the meantime, make the frosting. Beat the butter and mascarpone cheese until creamy. Add in the melted chocolate chips and vanilla paste.

6. Gradually, stir in the confectioner's swerve and salt; beat until everything's well combined. Lastly, frost the brownies and serve.

522.Blueberry & Lemon Cake

Servings:4
Cooking Time: 17 Minutes
Ingredients:
- 2 eggs
- 1 cup blueberries
- zest from 1 lemon
- juice from 1 lemon
- 1 tsp. vanilla
- brown sugar for topping (a little sprinkling on top of each muffin-less than a teaspoon)
- 2 1/2 cups self-rising flour
- 1/2 cup Monk Fruit (or use your preferred sugar)
- 1/2 cup cream
- 1/4 cup avocado oil (any light cooking oil)

Directions:
1. In mixing bowl, beat well wet Ingredients. Stir in dry ingredients and mix thoroughly.
2. Lightly grease baking pan of air fryer with cooking spray. Pour in batter.
3. For 12 minutes, cook on 330 °F.
4. Let it stand in air fryer for 5 minutes.
5. Serve and enjoy.

523.Flavorsome Peach Cake

Servings:6
Cooking Time:40 Minutes
Ingredients:
- 1/2 pound peaches, pitted and mashed
- 3 tablespoons honey
- 1/2 teaspoon baking powder
- 1 ¼ cups cake flour
- 1/2 teaspoon orange extract
- 1 teaspoon pure vanilla extract
- 1/4 teaspoon ground cinnamon
- 1/3 cup ghee
- 1/8 teaspoon salt
- 1/2 cup caster sugar
- 2 eggs
- 1/4 teaspoon freshly grated nutmeg

Directions:
1. Firstly, preheat the air fryer to 310 degrees F. Spritz the cake pan with a nonstick cooking spray.
2. In a mixing bowl, beat the ghee with caster sugar until creamy. Fold in the egg, mashed peaches and honey.
3. Then, make the cake batter by mixing the remaining ingredients; now, stir in the peach/honey mixture.
4. Now, transfer the prepared batter to the cake pan; level the surface with a spoon.

5. Bake for 35 minutes or until a tester inserted in the center of your cake comes out completely dry. Enjoy!

524.Cream Doughnuts

Servings:8
Cooking Time:16 Minutes
Ingredients:
- 4 tablespoons butter, softened and divided
- 2 egg yolks
- 2¼ cups plain flour
- 1½ teaspoons baking powder
- ½ cup sugar
- 1 teaspoon salt
- ½ cup sour cream
- ½ cup heavy cream

Directions:
1. Preheat the Air fryer to 355 °F and grease an Air fryer basket lightly.
2. Sift together flour, baking powder and salt in a large bowl.
3. Add sugar and cold butter and mix until a coarse crumb is formed.
4. Stir in the egg yolks, ½ of the sour cream and 1/3 of the flour mixture and mix until a dough is formed.
5. Add remaining sour cream and 1/3 of the flour mixture and mix until well combined.
6. Stir in the remaining flour mixture and combine well.
7. Roll the dough into ½ inch thickness onto a floured surface and cut into donuts with a donut cutter.
8. Coat butter on both sides of the donuts and arrange in the Air fryer basket.
9. Cook for about 8 minutes until golden and top with heavy cream to serve.

525.Coconut Chip Cookies

Servings: 12
Cooking Time: 20 Minutes
Ingredients:
- 1 cup butter, melted
- 1 ¾ cups granulated sugar
- 3 eggs
- 2 tablespoons coconut milk
- 1 teaspoon coconut extract
- 1 teaspoon vanilla extract
- 2 ¼ cups all-purpose flour
- 1/2 teaspoon baking powder
- 1/2 teaspoon baking soda
- 1/2 teaspoon fine table salt
- 2 cups coconut chips

Directions:
1. Begin by preheating your Air Fryer to 350 degrees F.
2. In the bowl of an electric mixer, beat the butter and sugar until well combined. Now, add the eggs one at a time, and mix well;

add the coconut milk, coconut extract, and vanilla; beat until creamy and uniform.
3. Mix the flour with baking powder, baking soda, and salt. Then, stir the flour mixture into the butter mixture and stir until everything is well incorporated.
4. Finally, fold in the coconut chips and mix again. Scoop out 1 tablespoon size balls of the batter on a cookie pan, leaving 2 inches between each cookie.
5. Bake for 10 minutes or until golden brown, rotating the pan once or twice through the cooking time.
6. Let your cookies cool on wire racks. Bon appétit!

526.Perfect Apple Pie

Servings:6
Cooking Time:30 Minutes
Ingredients:
- 1 frozen pie crust, thawed
- 1 large apple, peeled, cored and chopped
- 1 tablespoon butter, chopped
- 1 egg, beaten
- 3 tablespoons sugar, divided
- 1 tablespoon ground cinnamon
- 2 teaspoons fresh lemon juice
- ½ teaspoon vanilla extract

Directions:
1. Preheat the Air fryer to 320 °F and grease a pie pan lightly.
2. Cut 2 crusts, first about 1/8-inch larger than pie pan and second, a little smaller than first one.
3. Arrange the large crust in the bottom of pie pan.
4. Mix apple, 2 tablespoons of sugar, cinnamon, lemon juice and vanilla extract in a large bowl.
5. Put the apple mixture evenly over the bottom crust and top with butter.
6. Arrange the second crust on top and seal the edges.
7. Cut 4 slits in the top crust carefully and brush with egg.
8. Sprinkle with sugar and arrange the pie pan in the Air fryer basket.
9. Cook for about 30 minutes and dish out to serve.

527.Cocoa Cupcakes

Servings: 4
Cooking Time: 25 Minutes
Ingredients:
- 1/3 cup coconut flour
- ½ cup cocoa powder
- 3 tablespoons stevia
- ½ teaspoon baking soda
- 1 teaspoon baking powder

- 4 eggs, whisked
- 1 teaspoon vanilla extract
- 4 tablespoons coconut oil, melted
- ¼ cup almond milk
- Cooking spray

Directions:
1. In a bowl, mix all the ingredients except the cooking spray and whisk well. Grease a cupcake tin that fits the air fryer with the cooking spray, pour the cupcake mix, put the pan in your air fryer, cook at 350 degrees F for 25 minutes, cool down and serve.

528.Classic Pound Cake

Servings: 8
Cooking Time: 35 Minutes
Ingredients:
- 1 stick butter, at room temperature
- 1 cup swerve
- 4 eggs
- 1 ½ cups coconut flour
- 1/2 teaspoon baking powder
- 1/2 teaspoon baking soda
- 1/4 teaspoon salt
- A pinch of freshly grated nutmeg
- A pinch of ground star anise
- 1/2 cup buttermilk
- 1 teaspoon vanilla essence

Directions:
1. Begin by preheating your Air Fryer to 320 degrees F. Spritz the bottom and sides of a baking pan with cooking spray.
2. Beat the butter and swerve with a hand mixer until creamy. Then, fold in the eggs, one at a time, and mix well until fluffy.
3. Stir in the flour along with the remaining ingredients. Mix to combine well. Scrape the batter into the prepared baking pan.
4. Bake for 15 minutes; rotate the pan and bake an additional 15 minutes, until the top of the cake springs back when gently pressed with your fingers. Bon appétit!

529.Ciabatta Chocolate Bread Pudding

Servings:6
Cooking Time:1 Hour
Ingredients:
- 3/4 cup chocolate chips morsels
- 2 teaspoons rum
- 8 slices ciabatta bread, cubed
- 1/3 cup coconut milk creamer
- 1/3 teaspoon ground cloves
- 3/4 cup turbinado sugar
- 3 ½ tablespoons coconut oil, room temperature
- 1 teaspoon candied ginger
- 2 eggs plus 1 egg yolk, lightly beaten
- 1 cup soy milk

Directions:
1. Grab two mixing dishes. Place cubed bread in the first dish.
2. In the second mixing dish, thoroughly combine the remaining ingredients; mix until everything is well combined.
3. Scrape the chocolate mix into the first dish with bread cubes. Allow it to soak for about 20 minutes. Evenly divide the mixture between 2 mini loaf pans.
4. Set the timer for 35 minutes. Bake in the preheated air fryer at 305 degrees F. Serve with whipped cream.Bon appétit!

530.Poppy Seed Pound Cake

Servings:8
Cooking Time: 20 Minutes
Ingredients:
- ¼ cup erythritol powder
- ¼ teaspoon vanilla extract
- ½ cup coconut milk
- 1 ½ cups almond flour
- 1 ½ teaspoon baking powder
- 1/3 cup butter, unsalted
- 2 large eggs, beaten
- 2 tablespoon psyllium husk powder
- 2 tablespoons poppy seeds

Directions:
1. Preheat the air fryer for 5 minutes.
2. In a mixing bowl, combine all ingredients.
3. Use a hand mixer to mix everything.
4. Pour into a small loaf pan that will fit in the air fryer.
5. Bake for 20 minutes at 375°F or until a toothpick inserted in the middle comes out clean.

531.Cranberry Jam

Servings: 8
Cooking Time: 20 Minutes
Ingredients:
- 2 pounds cranberries
- 4 ounces black currant
- 2 pounds sugar
- Zest of 1 lime
- 3 tablespoons water

Directions:
1. In a pan that fits your air fryer, add all the ingredients and stir.
2. Place the pan in the fryer and cook at 360 degrees F for 20 minutes.
3. Stir the jam well, divide into cups, refrigerate, and serve cold.

532.Mini Almond Cakes

Servings: 4
Cooking Time: 20 Minutes
Ingredients:
- 3 ounces dark chocolate, melted

- ¼ cup coconut oil, melted
- 2 tablespoons swerve
- 2 eggs, whisked
- ¼ teaspoon vanilla extract
- 1 tablespoon almond flour
- Cooking spray

Directions:
1. In bowl, combine all the ingredients except the cooking spray and whisk really well. Divide this into 4 ramekins greased with cooking spray, put them in the fryer and cook at 360 degrees F for 20 minutes. Serve warm.

533.Chocolate Cheesecake

Servings: 4
Cooking Time: 60 Minutes
Ingredients:
- 4 oz cream cheese
- ½ oz heavy cream
- 1 tsp Sugar Glycerite
- 1 tsp Splenda
- 1 oz Enjoy Life mini chocolate chips

Directions:
1. Combine all the ingredients except the chocolate to a thick consistency.
2. Fold in the chocolate chips.
3. Refrigerate in serving cups.
4. Serve!

534.Chocolate Balls

Servings:8
Cooking Time:13 Minutes
Ingredients:
- 2 cups plain flour
- 2 tablespoons cocoa powder
- ¾ cup chilled butter
- ¼ cup chocolate, chopped into 8 chunks
- ½ cup icing sugar
- Pinch of ground cinnamon
- 1 teaspoon vanilla extract

Directions:
1. Preheat the Air fryer to 355 °F and grease a baking dish lightly.
2. Mix flour, icing sugar, cocoa powder, cinnamon and vanilla extract in a bowl.
3. Add cold butter and buttermilk and mix until a smooth dough is formed.
4. Divide the dough into 8 equal balls and press 1 chocolate chunk in the center of each ball.
5. Cover completely with the dough and arrange the balls in a baking dish.
6. Transfer into the Air fryer and cook for about 8 minutes.
7. Set the Air fryer to 320 °F and cook for 5 more minutes.
8. Dish out in a platter and serve to enjoy.

535.Strawberry Shake

Servings: 1
Cooking Time: 5 Minutes
Ingredients:
- 3/4 cup coconut milk (from the carton)
- ¼ cup heavy cream
- 7 ice cubes
- 2 tbsp sugar-free strawberry Torani syrup
- ¼ tsp Xanthan Gum

Directions:
1. Combine all the ingredients into blender.
2. Blend for 1-2 minutes.
3. Serve!

536.Chocolate Yogurt Pecans Muffins

Servings:9
Cooking Time:10 Minutes
Ingredients:
- 1½ cups all-purpose flour
- 2 teaspoons baking powder
- 1 cup yogurt
- ¼ cup mini chocolate chips
- ¼ cup pecans, chopped
- ¼ cup sugar
- ½ teaspoon salt
- 1/3 cup vegetable oil
- 2 teaspoons vanilla extract

Directions:
1. Preheat the Air fryer to 355 °F and grease 9 muffin molds lightly.
2. Mix flour, sugar, baking powder, and salt in a bowl.
3. Mix the yogurt, oil, and vanilla extract in another bowl.
4. Fold in the chocolate chips and pecans and divide the mixture evenly into the muffin molds.
5. Arrange the muffin molds into the Air fryer basket and cook for about 10 minutes.
6. Remove the muffin molds from Air fryer and invert the muffins onto wire rack to cool completely before serving.

537.Clove Crackers

Servings: 8
Cooking Time: 33 Minutes
Ingredients:
- 1 cup almond flour
- 1 teaspoon xanthan gum
- 1 teaspoon flax meal
- ½ teaspoon salt
- 1 teaspoon baking powder
- 1 teaspoon lemon juice
- ½ teaspoon ground clove
- 2 tablespoons Erythritol
- 1 egg, beaten
- 3 tablespoons coconut oil, softened

Directions:

1. In the mixing bowl mix up almond flour, xanthan gum, flax meal, salt, baking powder, and ground clove. Add Erythritol, lemon juice, egg, and coconut oil. Stir the mixture gently with the help of the fork. Then knead the mixture till you get a soft dough. Line the chopping board with parchment. Put the dough on the parchment and roll it up in a thin layer. Cut the thin dough into squares (crackers). Preheat the air fryer to 360F. Line the air fryer basket with baking paper. Put the prepared crackers in the air fryer basket in one layer and cook them for 11 minutes or until the crackers are dry and light brown. Repeat the same steps with remaining uncooked crackers.

538.Speedy Chocolate Cookie

Servings:4
Cooking Time: 15 Minutes
Ingredients:
- 1 cup flour
- ¼ tsp baking powder
- 1/8 tsp salt
- ¼ cup sugar
- ¼ cup unsalted butter, softened
- 1 egg yolk
- ½ tsp vanilla extract
- ½ cup dark chocolate chips

Directions:
1. Preheat the Air fryer to 360 F. Line the air fryer basket with parchment paper.
2. In a bowl, sift flour with baking powder and salt. In another bowl, combine sugar, butter, and honey; stir in egg yolk and vanilla until everything is well incorporated. Add in the dry ingredients until mixed. Fold in chocolate chips.
3. Spread the batter on the bottom of the air fryer basket and cook for 8 minutes until just set. Allow to cool on a wire rack and serve.

539.Lemon Cheesecake

Servings:8
Cooking Time: 25 Minutes
Ingredients:
- 17.6 ounces ricotta cheese
- 3 eggs
- ¾ cup sugar
- 3 tablespoons corn starch
- 1 tablespoon fresh lemon juice
- 2 teaspoons vanilla extract
- 1 teaspoon fresh lemon zest, finely grated

Directions:
1. In a large bowl, put all ingredients and mix until well combined.
2. Place the mixture into a baking dish.

3. Set the temperature of air fryer to 320 degrees F.
4. Arrange the baking dish into an air fryer basket.
5. Air fry for about 25 minutes.
6. Remove from the air fryer and set aside for about 1-2 hours to cool.
7. Refrigerate to chill for about 2-3 hours before serving.

540.Super Moist Chocolate Cake

Servings:9
Cooking Time:40 Minutes
Ingredients:
- 1/3 cup plain flour
- ¼ teaspoon baking powder
- 1½ tablespoons unsweetened cocoa powder
- 2 eggs, yolks and whites separated
- 3¾ tablespoons milk
- 1½-ounce castor sugar, divided
- 2 tablespoon vegetable oil
- 1 teaspoon vanilla extract
- 1/8 teaspoon cream of tartar

Directions:
1. Preheat the Air fryer to 330 °F and grease a chiffon pan lightly.
2. Mix flour, baking powder and cocoa powder in a bowl.
3. Combine the remaining ingredients in another bowl until well combined.
4. Stir in the flour mixture slowly and pour this mixture into the chiffon pan.
5. Cover with the foil paper and poke some holes in the foil paper.
6. Transfer the baking pan into the Air fryer basket and cook for about 30 minutes.
7. Remove the foil and set the Air fryer to 285 °F.
8. Cook for 10 more minutes and cut into slices to serve.

541.Brownies

Servings: 6
Cooking Time: 25 Minutes
Ingredients:
- 6 tablespoons cream cheese, soft
- 3 eggs, whisked
- 2 tablespoons cocoa powder
- 3 tablespoons coconut oil, melted
- ¼ cup almond flour
- ¼ cup coconut flour
- ¼ teaspoon baking soda
- 1 teaspoon vanilla extract
- ½ cup almond milk
- 3 tablespoons swerve
- Cooking spray

Directions:

1. Grease a cake pan that fits the air fryer with the cooking spray. In a bowl, mix rest of the ingredients, whisk well and pour into the pan. Put the pan in your air fryer, cook at 370 degrees F for 25 minutes, cool the brownies down, slice and serve.

542.Homemade Coconut Banana Treat

Servings: 6
Cooking Time: 20 Minutes
Ingredients:
- 2 tbsp. coconut oil
- ¾ cup friendly bread crumbs
- 2 tbsp. sugar
- ½ tsp. cinnamon powder
- ¼ tsp. ground cloves
- 6 ripe bananas, peeled and halved
- ⅓ cup flour
- 1 large egg, beaten

Directions:
1. Heat a skillet over a medium heat. Add in the coconut oil and the bread crumbs, and mix together for approximately 4 minutes.
2. Take the skillet off of the heat.
3. Add in the sugar, cinnamon, and cloves.
4. Cover all sides of the banana halves with the rice flour.
5. Dip each one in the beaten egg before coating them in the bread crumb mix.
6. Place the banana halves in the Air Fryer basket, taking care not to overlap them. Cook at 290°F for 10 minutes. You may need to complete this step in multiple batches.
7. Serve hot or at room temperature, topped with a sprinkling of flaked coconut if desired.

543.Air Fried Apricots In Whiskey Sauce

Servings:4
Cooking Time:45 Minutes
Ingredients:
- 1 pound apricot, pitted and halved
- 1/4 cup whiskey
- 1 teaspoon pure vanilla extract
- 1/2 stick butter, room temperature
- 2-4 whole cloves
- 1 cup cool whip, for serving
- 1/2 cup maple syrup

Directions:
1. In a small-sized saucepan that is placed over a moderate flame, heat the maple syrup, vanilla, and butter; simmer until the butter has melted.
2. Add the whiskey and stir to combine. Arrange the apricots wedges on the bottom of a lightly greased baking dish.

3. Pour the sauce over the apricots; scatter whole cloves over the top. Then, transfer the baking dish to the preheated air fryer.
4. Air-fryer at 380 degrees F for 35 minutes. Top with cool whip and serve. Bon appétit!

544.Fruity Oreo Muffins

Servings:6
Cooking Time:10 Minutes
Ingredients:
- 1 cup milk
- 1 pack Oreo biscuits, crushed
- ¾ teaspoon baking powder
- 1 banana, peeled and chopped
- 1 apple, peeled, cored and chopped
- 1 teaspoon cocoa powder
- 1 teaspoon honey
- 1 teaspoon fresh lemon juice
- A pinch of ground cinnamon

Directions:
1. Preheat the Air fryer to 320 °F and grease 6 muffin cups lightly.
2. Mix milk, biscuits, cocoa powder, baking soda, and baking powder in a bowl until well combined.
3. Transfer the mixture into the muffin cups and cook for about 10 minutes.
4. Remove from the Air fryer and invert the muffin cups onto a wire rack to cool.
5. Meanwhile, mix the banana, apple, honey, lemon juice, and cinnamon in another bowl.
6. Scoop some portion of muffins from the center and fill with fruit mixture to serve.

545.Coffee Surprise

Servings: 1
Cooking Time: 5 Minutes
Ingredients:
- 2 heaped tbsp flaxseed, ground
- 100ml cooking cream 35% fat
- ½ tsp cocoa powder, dark and unsweetened
- 1 tbsp goji berries
- Freshly brewed coffee

Directions:
1. Mix together the flaxseeds, cream and cocoa and coffee.
2. Season with goji berries.
3. Serve!

546.Strawberry Cupcakes

Servings:10
Cooking Time:8 Minutes
Ingredients:
- For Cupcakes:
- 7 tablespoons butter
- 2 eggs
- 7/8 cup self-rising flour
- For Icing:
- 3½ tablespoons butter

- ¼ cup fresh strawberries, blended
- For Cupcakes:
- ½ cup caster sugar
- ½ teaspoon vanilla essence
- For Icing:
- 1 cup icing sugar
- 1 tablespoon whipped cream
- ½ teaspoon pink food color

Directions:
1. Preheat the Air fryer to 340 °F and grease 8 muffin tins lightly.
2. For Cupcakes:
3. Mix all the ingredients in a large bowl until well combined.
4. Transfer the mixture into muffin tins and place in the Air fryer basket.
5. Cook for about 8 minutes and dish out.
6. For Icing:
7. Mix all the ingredients in a large bowl until well combined.
8. Fill the pastry bag with icing and top each cupcake evenly with frosting to serve.

547.Fried Banana Slices

Servings:8
Cooking Time:15 Minutes
Ingredients:
- 4 medium ripe bananas, peeled and cut in 4 pieces lengthwise
- 1/3 cup rice flour, divided
- 4 tablespoons corn flour
- 2 tablespoons desiccated coconut
- ½ teaspoon baking powder
- ½ teaspoon ground cardamom
- A pinch of salt

Directions:
1. Preheat the Air fryer to 390 °F and grease an Air fryer basket.
2. Mix coconut, 2 tablespoons of rice flour, corn flour, baking powder, cardamom, and salt in a shallow bowl.
3. Stir in the water gradually and mix until a smooth mixture is formed.
4. Place the remaining rice flour in a second bowl and dip in the coconut mixture.
5. Dredge in the rice flour and arrange the banana slices into the Air fryer basket in a single layer.
6. Cook for about 15 minutes, flipping once in between and dish out onto plates to serve.

548.Ricotta Cheese Cake

Servings: 8
Cooking Time: 30 Minutes
Ingredients:
- 3 eggs, lightly beaten
- 1 tsp baking powder
- ½ cup ghee, melted
- 1 cup almond flour

- 1/3 cup erythritol
- 1 cup ricotta cheese, soft

Directions:
1. Add all ingredients into the bowl and mix until well combined.
2. Pour batter into the greased air fryer baking dish and place into the air fryer.
3. Cook at 350 F for 30 minutes.
4. Slice and serve.

549.Sugar Butter Fritters

Servings: 16
Cooking Time: 30 Minutes
Ingredients:
- For the dough:
- 4 cups flour
- 1 tsp. kosher salt
- 1 tsp. sugar
- 3 tbsp. butter, at room temperature
- 1 packet instant yeast
- 1 ¼ cups lukewarm water
- For the Cakes
- 1 cup sugar
- Pinch of cardamom

- 1 tsp. cinnamon powder
- 1 stick butter, melted

Directions:
1. Place all of the ingredients in a large bowl and combine well.
2. Add in the lukewarm water and mix until a soft, elastic dough forms.
3. Place the dough on a lightly floured surface and lay a greased sheet of aluminum foil on top of the dough. Refrigerate for 5 to 10 minutes.
4. Remove it from the refrigerator and divide it in two. Mold each half into a log and slice it into 20 pieces.
5. In a shallow bowl, combine the sugar, cardamom and cinnamon.
6. Coat the slices with a light brushing of melted butter and the sugar.
7. Spritz Air Fryer basket with cooking spray.
8. Transfer the slices to the fryer and air fry at 360°F for roughly 10 minutes. Turn each slice once during the baking time.
9. Dust each slice with the sugar before serving.

OTHER AIR FRYER RECIPES

550.Fluffy Omelet With Leftover Beef

Servings: 4
Cooking Time: 20 Minutes
Ingredients:
- Non-stick cooking spray
- 1/2 pound leftover beef, coarsely chopped
- 2 garlic cloves, pressed
- 1 cup kale, torn into pieces and wilted
- 1 bell pepper, chopped
- 6 eggs, beaten
- 6 tablespoons sour cream
- 1/2 teaspoon turmeric powder
- 1 teaspoon red pepper flakes
- Salt and ground black pepper, to your liking

Directions:
1. Spritz the inside of four ramekins with a cooking spray.
2. Divide all of the above ingredients among the prepared ramekins. Stir until everything is well combined.
3. Air-fry at 360 degrees F for 16 minutes; check with a wooden stick and return the eggs to the Air Fryer for a few more minutes as needed. Serve immediately.

551.Cheese And Garlic Stuffed Chicken Breasts

Servings: 2
Cooking Time: 20 Minutes
Ingredients:
- 1/2 cup Cottage cheese
- 2 eggs, beaten
- 2 medium-sized chicken breasts, halved
- 2 tablespoons fresh coriander, chopped
- 1teaspoon fine sea salt
- Seasoned breadcrumbs
- 1/3teaspoon freshly ground black pepper, to savor
- 3 cloves garlic, finely minced

Directions:
1. Firstly, flatten out the chicken breast using a meat tenderizer.
2. In a medium-sized mixing dish, combine the Cottage cheese with the garlic, coriander, salt, and black pepper.
3. Spread 1/3 of the mixture over the first chicken breast. Repeat with the remaining ingredients. Roll the chicken around the filling; make sure to secure with toothpicks.
4. Now, whisk the egg in a shallow bowl. In another shallow bowl, combine the salt, ground black pepper, and seasoned breadcrumbs.
5. Coat the chicken breasts with the whisked egg; now, roll them in the breadcrumbs.

6. Cook in the air fryer cooking basket at 365 degrees F for 22 minutes. Serve immediately.

552.Rosemary Roasted Mixed Nuts

Servings: 6
Cooking Time: 20 Minutes
Ingredients:
- 2 tablespoons butter, at room temperature
- 1 tablespoon dried rosemary
- 1 teaspoon coarse sea salt
- 1/2 teaspoon paprika
- 1/2 cup pine nuts
- 1 cup pecans
- 1/2 cup hazelnuts

Directions:
1. Toss all the ingredients in the mixing bowl.
2. Line the Air Fryer basket with baking parchment. Spread out the coated nuts in a single layer in the basket.
3. Roast at 350 degrees F for 6 to 8 minutes, shaking the basket once or twice. Work in batches. Enjoy!

553.Za'atar Eggs With Chicken And Provolone Cheese

Servings: 2
Cooking Time: 20 Minutes
Ingredients:
- 1/3 cup milk
- 1 1/2 Roma tomato, chopped
- 1/3 cup Provolone cheese, grated
- 1 teaspoon freshly cracked pink peppercorns
- 3 eggs
- 1 teaspoon Za'atar
- ½ chicken breast, cooked
- 1 teaspoon fine sea salt
- 1 teaspoon freshly cracked pink peppercorns

Directions:
1. Preheat your air fryer to cook at 365 degrees F. In a medium-sized mixing dish, whisk the eggs together with the milk, Za'atar, sea salt, and cracked pink peppercorns.
2. Spritz the ramekins with cooking oil; divide the prepared egg mixture among the greased ramekins.
3. Shred the chicken with two forks or a stand mixer. Add the shredded chicken to the ramekins, followed by the tomato and the cheese.
4. To finish, air-fry for 18 minutes or until it is done. Bon appétit!

554. Cottage Cheese Stuffed Chicken Rolls

Servings: 2
Cooking Time: 20 Minutes
Ingredients:
- 1/2 cup Cottage cheese
- 2 eggs, beaten
- 2 medium-sized chicken breasts, halved
- 2 tablespoons fresh coriander, chopped
- 1 teaspoon fine sea salt
- 1/2 cup parmesan cheese, grated
- 1/3 teaspoon freshly ground black pepper, to savor
- 3 cloves garlic, finely minced

Directions:
1. Firstly, flatten out the chicken breast using a meat tenderizer.
2. In a medium-sized mixing dish, combine the Cottage cheese with the garlic, coriander, salt, and black pepper.
3. Spread 1/3 of the mixture over the first chicken breast. Repeat with the remaining ingredients. Roll the chicken around the filling; make sure to secure with toothpicks.
4. Now, whisk the egg in a shallow bowl. In another shallow bowl, combine the salt, ground black pepper, and parmesan cheese.
5. Coat the chicken breasts with the whisked egg; now, roll them in the parmesan cheese.
6. Cook in the air fryer cooking basket at 365 degrees F for 22 minutes. Serve immediately.

555. Dijon And Curry Turkey Cutlets

Servings: 4
Cooking Time: 30 Minutes + Marinating Time
Ingredients:
- 1/2 tablespoon Dijon mustard
- 1/2 teaspoon curry powder
- Sea salt flakes and freshly cracked black peppercorns, to savor
- 1/3 pound turkey cutlets
- 1/2 cup fresh lemon juice
- 1/2 tablespoons tamari sauce

Directions:
1. Set the air fryer to cook at 375 degrees. Then, put the turkey cutlets into a mixing dish; add fresh lemon juice, tamari, and mustard; let it marinate at least 2 hours.
2. Coat each turkey cutlet with the curry powder, salt, and freshly cracked black peppercorns; roast for 28 minutes; work in batches. Bon appétit!

556. Two Cheese And Shrimp Dip

Servings: 8
Cooking Time: 25 Minutes
Ingredients:
- 2 teaspoons butter, melted
- 8 ounces shrimp, peeled and deveined
- 2 garlic cloves, minced
- 1/4 cup chicken stock
- 2 tablespoons fresh lemon juice
- Salt and ground black pepper, to taste
- 1/2 teaspoon red pepper flakes
- 4 ounces cream cheese, at room temperature
- 1/2 cup sour cream
- 4 tablespoons mayonnaise
- 1/4 cup mozzarella cheese, shredded

Directions:
1. Start by preheating the Air Fryer to 395 degrees F. Grease the sides and bottom of a baking dish with the melted butter.
2. Place the shrimp, garlic, chicken stock, lemon juice, salt, black pepper, and red pepper flakes in the baking dish.
3. Transfer the baking dish to the cooking basket and bake for 10 minutes. Add the mixture to your food processor; pulse until the coarsely is chopped.
4. Add the cream cheese, sour cream, and mayonnaise. Top with the mozzarella cheese and bake in the preheated Air Fryer at 360 degrees F for 6 to 7 minutes or until the cheese is bubbling.
5. Serve immediately with breadsticks if desired. Bon appétit!

557. Omelet With Smoked Tofu And Veggies

Servings: 2
Cooking Time: 20 Minutes
Ingredients:
- 2 eggs, beaten
- 1/3 cup cherry tomatoes, chopped
- 1 bell pepper, seeded and chopped
- 1/3 teaspoon freshly ground black pepper
- 1/2 purple onion, peeled and sliced
- 1 teaspoon smoked cayenne pepper
- 5 medium-sized eggs, well-beaten
- 1/3 cup smoked tofu, crumbled
- 1 teaspoon seasoned salt
- 1 1/2 tablespoons fresh chives, chopped

Directions:
1. Brush a baking dish with a spray coating.
2. Throw all ingredients, minus fresh chives, into the baking dish; give it a good stir.
3. Cook about 15 minutes at 325 degrees F. Garnish with fresh chopped chives. Bon appétit!

558. Baked Eggs With Linguica Sausage

Servings: 2
Cooking Time: 18 Minutes
Ingredients:
- 1/2 cup Cheddar cheese, shredded
- 4 eggs

- 2 ounces Linguica (Portuguese pork sausage), chopped
- 1/2 onion, peeled and chopped
- 2 tablespoons olive oil
- 1/2 teaspoon rosemary, chopped
- ½ teaspoon marjoram
- 1/4 cup sour cream
- Sea salt and freshly ground black pepper, to taste
- ½ teaspoon fresh sage, chopped

Directions:
1. Lightly grease 2 oven safe ramekins with olive oil. Now, divide the sausage and onions among these ramekins.
2. Crack an egg into each ramekin; add the remaining items, minus the cheese. Air-fry at 355 degrees F approximately 13 minutes.
3. Immediately top with Cheddar cheese, serve, and enjoy.

559.Easy Pork Burgers With Blue Cheese

Servings: 6
Cooking Time: 44 Minutes
Ingredients:
- 1/3 cup blue cheese, crumbled
- 6 hamburger buns, toasted
- 2 teaspoons dried basil
- 1/3 teaspoon smoked paprika
- 1 pound ground pork
- 2 tablespoons tomato puree
- 2 small-sized onions, peeled and chopped
- 1/2 teaspoon ground black pepper
- 3 garlic cloves, minced
- 1 teaspoon fine sea salt

Directions:
1. Start by preheating your air fryer to 385 degrees F.
2. In a mixing dish, combine the pork, onion, garlic, tomato puree, and seasonings; mix to combine well.
3. Form the pork mixture into six patties; cook the burgers for 23 minutes. Pause the machine, turn the temperature to 365 degrees F and cook for 18 more minutes.
4. Place the prepared burger on the bottom bun; top with blue cheese; assemble the burgers and serve warm.

560.Oatmeal Pizza Cups

Servings: 4
Cooking Time: 30 Minutes
Ingredients:
- 1 cup rolled oats
- 1 teaspoon baking powder
- 1/4 teaspoon ground black pepper
- Salt, to taste
- 2 tablespoons butter, melted
- 1 cup milk
- 4 slices smoked ham, chopped

- 4 ounces mozzarella cheese, shredded
- 4 tablespoons ketchup

Directions:
1. Start by preheating your Air Fryer to 350 degrees F. Now, lightly grease a muffin tin with nonstick spray.
2. Pulse the rolled oats, baking powder, pepper, and salt in your food processor until the mixture looks like coarse meal.
3. Add the remaining ingredients and stir to combine well. Spoon the mixture into the prepared muffin tin.
4. Bake in the preheated Air Fryer for 20 minutes until a toothpick inserted comes out clean. Bon appétit!

561.Egg Salad With Asparagus And Spinach

Servings: 4
Cooking Time: 25 Minutes + Chilling Time
Ingredients:
- 4 eggs
- 1 pound asparagus, chopped
- 2 cup baby spinach
- 1/2 cup mayonnaise
- 1 teaspoon mustard
- 1 teaspoon fresh lemon juice
- Sea salt and ground black pepper, to taste

Directions:
1. Place the wire rack in the Air Fryer basket; lower the eggs onto the wire rack.
2. Cook at 270 degrees F for 15 minutes.
3. Transfer them to an ice-cold water bath to stop the cooking. Peel the eggs under cold running water; coarsely chop the hard-boiled eggs and set aside.
4. Increase the temperature to 400 degrees F. Place your asparagus in the lightly greased Air Fryer basket.
5. Cook for 5 minutes or until tender. Place in a nice salad bowl. Add the baby spinach.
6. In a mixing dish, thoroughly combine the remaining ingredients. Drizzle this dressing over the asparagus in the salad bowl and top with the chopped eggs. Bon appétit!

562.The Best London Broil Ever

Servings: 8
Cooking Time: 30 Minutes + Marinating Time
Ingredients:
- 2 pounds London broil
- 3 large garlic cloves, minced
- 3 tablespoons balsamic vinegar
- 3 tablespoons whole-grain mustard
- 2 tablespoons olive oil
- Sea salt and ground black pepper, to taste
- 1/2 teaspoon dried hot red pepper flakes

Directions:
1. Score both sides of the cleaned London broil.

2. Thoroughly combine the remaining ingredients; massage this mixture into the meat to coat it on all sides. Let it marinate for at least 3 hours.
3. Set the Air Fryer to cook at 400 degrees F; Then cook the London broil for 15 minutes. Flip it over and cook another 10 to 12 minutes. Bon appétit!

563. Breakfast Muffins With Mushrooms And Goat Cheese

Servings: 6
Cooking Time: 25 Minutes
Ingredients:
- 2 tablespoons butter, melted
- 1 yellow onion, chopped
- 2 garlic cloves, minced
- 1 cup brown mushrooms, sliced
- Sea salt and ground black pepper, to taste
- 1 teaspoon fresh basil
- 8 eggs, lightly whisked
- 6 tablespoons goat cheese, crumbled

Directions:
1. Start by preheating your Air Fryer to 330 degrees F. Now, spritz a 6-tin muffin tin with cooking spray.
2. Melt the butter in a heavy-bottomed skillet over medium-high heat. Sauté the onions, garlic, and mushrooms until just tender and fragrant.
3. Add the salt, black pepper, and basil and remove from heat. Divide out the sautéed mixture into the muffin tin.
4. Pour the whisked eggs on top and top with the goat cheese. Bake for 20 minutes rotating the pan halfway through the cooking time. Bon appétit!

564. Old-fashioned Beef Stroganoff

Servings: 4
Cooking Time: 20 Minutes
Ingredients:
- 3/4 pound beef sirloin steak, cut into small-sized strips
- 1/4 cup balsamic vinegar
- 1 tablespoon brown mustard
- 2 tablespoons all-purpose flour
- 1 tablespoon butter
- 1 cup beef broth
- 1 cup leek, chopped
- 2 cloves garlic, crushed
- 1 teaspoon cayenne pepper
- Sea salt flakes and crushed red pepper, to taste
- 1 cup sour cream
- 2 ½ tablespoons tomato paste

Directions:
1. Place the beef along with the balsamic vinegar and the mustard in a mixing dish;

cover and marinate in your refrigerator for about 1 hour.
2. Then, coat the beef strips with the flour; butter the inside of a baking dish and put the beef into the dish.
3. Add the broth, leeks and garlic. Cook at 380 degrees for 8 minutes. Pause the machine and add the cayenne pepper, salt, red pepper, sour cream and tomato paste; cook for additional 7 minutes.
4. Check for doneness and serve with warm egg noodles, if desired. Bon appétit!

565. Greek Frittata With Feta Cheese

Servings: 4
Cooking Time: 10 Minutes
Ingredients:
- 1/3 cup Feta cheese, crumbled
- 1 teaspoon dried rosemary
- 2 tablespoons fish sauce
- 1 ½ cup cooked chicken breasts, boneless and shredded
- 1/2 teaspoon coriander sprig, finely chopped
- 6 medium-sized whisked eggs
- 1/3 teaspoon ground white pepper
- 1 cup fresh chives, chopped
- 1/2 teaspoon garlic paste
- Fine sea salt, to taste
- Nonstick cooking spray

Directions:
1. Grab a baking dish that fit in your Air Fryer.
2. Lightly coat the inside of the baking dish with a nonstick cooking spray of choice. Stir in all ingredients, minus feta cheese. Stir to combine well.
3. Set your Air Fryer to cook at 335 degrees for 8 minutes; check for doneness. Scatter crumbled feta over the top and eat immediately!

566. Wine-braised Turkey Breasts

Servings: 4
Cooking Time: 30 Minutes + Marinating Time
Ingredients:
- 1/3 cup dry white wine
- 1½ tablespoon sesame oil
- 1/2 pound turkey breasts, boneless, skinless and sliced
- 1/2 tablespoon honey
- 1/2 cup plain flour
- 2 tablespoons oyster sauce
- Sea salt flakes and cracked black peppercorns, to taste

Directions:
1. Set the air fryer to cook at 385 degrees. Pat the turkey slices dry and season with the sea salt flakes and the cracked peppercorns.

2. In a bowl, mix the other ingredients together, minus the flour; rub your turkey with this mixture. Set aside to marinate for at least 55 minutes.
3. Coat each turkey slice with the plain flour. Cook for 27 minutes; make sure to flip once or twice and work in batches. Bon appétit!

567.Cheesy Zucchini With Queso Añejo

Servings: 4
Cooking Time: 25 Minutes
Ingredients:
- 1 large-sized zucchini, thinly sliced
- 1/4 cup almond flour
- 1 cup parmesan cheese
- 1 egg, whisked
- 1/2 cup Queso Añejo, grated
- Salt and cracked pepper, to taste

Directions:
1. Pat dry the zucchini slices with a kitchen towel.
2. Mix the remaining ingredients in a shallow bowl; mix until everything is well combined. Dip each zucchini slice in the prepared batter.
3. Cook in the preheated Air Fryer at 400 degrees F for 12 minutes, shaking the basket halfway through the cooking time.
4. Work in batches until the zucchini slices are crispy and golden brown. Enjoy!

568.Mother's Day Pudding

Servings: 6
Cooking Time: 45 Minutes
Ingredients:
- 1 pound French baguette bread, cubed
- 4 eggs, beaten
- 1/4 cup chocolate liqueur
- 1 cup granulated sugar
- 2 tablespoons honey
- 2 cups whole milk
- 1/2 cup heavy cream
- 1 teaspoon vanilla extract
- 1/4 teaspoon ground cloves
- 2 ounces milk chocolate chips

Directions:
1. Place the bread cubes in a lightly greased baking dish. In a mixing bowl, thoroughly combine the eggs, chocolate liqueur, sugar, honey, milk, heavy cream, vanilla, and ground cloves.
2. Pour the custard over the bread cubes. Scatter the milk chocolate chips over the top of your bread pudding.
3. Let stand for 30 minutes, occasionally pressing with a wide spatula to submerge.
4. Cook in the preheated Air Fryer at 370 degrees F degrees for 7 minutes; check to

ensure even cooking and cook an additional 5 to 6 minutes. Bon appétit!

569.Beef And Kale Omelet

Servings: 4
Cooking Time: 20 Minutes
Ingredients:
- Non-stick cooking spray
- 1/2 pound leftover beef, coarsely chopped
- 2 garlic cloves, pressed
- 1 cup kale, torn into pieces and wilted
- 1 tomato, chopped
- 1/4 teaspoon brown sugar
- 4 eggs, beaten
- 4 tablespoons heavy cream
- 1/2 teaspoon turmeric powder
- Salt and ground black pepper, to your liking
- 1/8 teaspoon ground allspice

Directions:
1. Spritz the inside of four ramekins with a cooking spray.
2. Divide all of the above ingredients among the prepared ramekins. Stir until everything is well combined.
3. Air-fry at 360 degrees F for 16 minutes; check with a wooden stick and return the eggs to the Air Fryer for a few more minutes as needed. Serve immediately.

570.Creamed Asparagus And Egg Salad

Servings: 4
Cooking Time: 25 Minutes + Chilling Time
Ingredients:
- 2 eggs
- 1 pound asparagus, chopped
- 2 cup baby spinach
- 1/2 cup mayonnaise
- 1 teaspoon mustard
- 1 teaspoon fresh lemon juice
- Sea salt and ground black pepper, to taste

Directions:
1. Place the wire rack in the Air Fryer basket; lower the eggs onto the wire rack.
2. Cook at 270 degrees F for 15 minutes.
3. Transfer them to an ice-cold water bath to stop the cooking. Peel the eggs under cold running water; coarsely chop the hard-boiled eggs and set aside.
4. Increase the temperature to 400 degrees F. Place your asparagus in the lightly greased Air Fryer basket.
5. Cook for 5 minutes or until tender. Place in a nice salad bowl. Add the baby spinach.
6. In a mixing dish, thoroughly combine the remaining ingredients. Drizzle this dressing over the asparagus in the salad bowl and top with the chopped eggs. Bon appétit!

571.Southwest Bean Potpie

Servings: 5
Cooking Time: 30 Minutes
Ingredients:
- 1 tablespoon olive oil
- 2 sweet peppers, seeded and sliced
- 1 carrot, chopped
- 1 onion, chopped
- 2 garlic cloves, minced
- 1 cup cooked bacon, diced
- 1 ½ cups beef bone broth
- 20 ounces canned red kidney beans, drained
- Sea salt and freshly ground black pepper, to taste
- 1 package (8 1/2-ounce) cornbread mix
- 1/2 cup milk
- 2 tablespoons butter, melted

Directions:
1. Heat the olive oil in a saucepan over medium-high heat. Now, cook the peppers, carrot, onion, and garlic until they have softened, about 7 minutes
2. Add the bacon and broth. Bring to a boil and cook for 2 minutes more. Stir in the kidney beans, salt and black pepper; continue to cook until everything is heated through.
3. Transfer the mixture to the lightly greased baking pan.
4. In a small bowl, combine the muffin mix, milk, and melted butter. Stir until well mixed and spoon evenly over the bean mixture. Smooth it with a spatula and transfer to the Air Fryer cooking basket.
5. Bake in the preheated Air Fryer at 400 degrees F for 12 minutes. Place on a wire rack to cool slightly before slicing and serving. Bon appétit!

572.Keto Brioche With Caciocavallo

Servings: 6
Cooking Time: 15 Minutes
Ingredients:
- 1/2 cup ricotta cheese, crumbled
- 1 cup part skim mozzarella cheese, shredded
- 1 egg
- 1/2 cup coconut flour
- 1/2 cup almond flour
- 1 teaspoon baking soda
- 2 tablespoons plain whey protein isolate
- 3 tablespoons sesame oil
- 2 teaspoons dried thyme
- 1 ½ cups Caciocavallo, grated
- 1 cup leftover chicken, shredded
- 3 eggs
- 1 teaspoon kosher salt
- 1 teaspoon freshly cracked black pepper, or more to taste
- 1/3 teaspoon gremolata

Directions:
1. To make the keto brioche, microwave the cheese for 1 minute 30 seconds, stirring twice. Add the cheese to the bowl of a food processor and blend well. Fold in the egg and mix again.
2. Add in the flour, baking soda, and plain whey protein isolate; blend again. Scrape the batter onto the center of a lightly greased cling film.
3. Form the dough into a disk and transfer to your freezer to cool; cut into 6 pieces and transfer to a parchment-lined baking pan (make sure to grease your hands).
4. Firstly, slice off the top of each brioche; then, scoop out the insides.
5. Brush each brioche with sesame oil. Add the remaining ingredients in the order listed above.
6. Place the prepared brioche onto the bottom of the cooking basket. Bake for 7 minutes at 345 degrees F. Bon appétit!

573.Brown Rice Bowl

Servings: 4
Cooking Time: 55 Minutes
Ingredients:
- 1 cup brown rice
- 1 tablespoon peanut oil
- 2 tablespoons soy sauce
- 1/2 cup scallions, chopped
- 2 bell pepper, chopped
- 2 eggs, beaten
- Sea salt and ground black pepper, to taste
- 1/2 teaspoon granulated garlic

Directions:
1. Heat the brown rice and 2 ½ cups of water in a saucepan over high heat. Bring it to a boil; turn the stove down to simmer and cook for 35 minutes.
2. Grease a baking pan with nonstick cooking spray. Add the hot rice and the other ingredients.
3. Cook at 370 degrees F for 15 minutes, checking occasionally to ensure even cooking. Enjoy!

574.Mini Bread Puddings With Cinnamon Glaze

Servings: 5
Cooking Time: 50 Minutes
Ingredients:
- 5 tablespoons butter
- 1/2 pound cinnamon-raisin bread, cubed
- 1 cup milk
- 1/2 cup double cream

- 2/3 cup sugar
- 1 tablespoon honey
- 1 teaspoon pure vanilla extract
- 2 eggs, lightly beaten
- Cinnamon Glaze:
- 1/4 cup powdered sugar
- 1 teaspoon ground cinnamon
- 1 tablespoon milk
- 1/2 teaspoon vanilla

Directions:
1. Begin by preheating your Air Fryer to 370 degrees F. Lightly butter five ramekins.
2. Place the bread cubes in the greased ramekins. In a mixing bowl, thoroughly combine the milk, double cream, sugar, honey, vanilla, and eggs.
3. Pour the custard over the bread cubes. Let it stand for 30 minutes, occasionally pressing with a wide spatula to submerge.
4. Cook in the preheated Air Fryer at 370 degrees F degrees for 7 minutes; check to ensure even cooking and cook an additional 5 to 6 minutes.
5. Meanwhile, prepare the glaze by whisking the powdered sugar, cinnamon, milk, and vanilla until smooth. Top the bread puddings with the glaze and serve at room temperature. Bon appétit!

575.Fingerling Potatoes With Cashew Sauce

Servings: 4
Cooking Time: 20 Minutes
Ingredients:
- 1 pound fingerling potatoes
- 1 tablespoon butter, melted
- Sea salt and ground black pepper, to your liking
- 1 teaspoon shallot powder
- 1 teaspoon garlic powder
- Cashew Sauce:
- 1/2 cup raw cashews
- 1 teaspoon cayenne pepper
- 3 tablespoons nutritional yeast
- 2 teaspoons white vinegar
- 4 tablespoons water
- 1/4 teaspoon dried rosemary
- 1/4 teaspoon dried dill

Directions:
1. Toss the potatoes with the butter, salt, black pepper, shallot powder, and garlic powder.
2. Place the fingerling potatoes in the lightly greased Air Fryer basket and cook at 400 degrees F for 6 minutes; shake the basket and cook for a further 6 minutes.
3. Meanwhile, make the sauce by mixing all ingredients in your food processor or high-speed blender.

4. Drizzle the cashew sauce over the potato wedges. Bake at 400 degrees F for 2 more minutes or until everything is heated through. Enjoy!

576.Grilled Cheese Sandwich

Servings: 1
Cooking Time: 15 Minutes
Ingredients:
- 2 slices artisan bread
- 1 tablespoon butter, softened
- 1 tablespoon tomato ketchup
- 1/2 teaspoon dried oregano
- 2 slices Cheddar cheese

Directions:
1. Brush one side of each slice of the bread with melted butter.
2. Add the tomato ketchup, oregano, and cheese. Make the sandwich and grill at 360 degrees F for 9 minutes or until cheese is melted. Bon appétit!

577.Japanese Fried Rice With Eggs

Servings: 2
Cooking Time: 30 Minutes
Ingredients:
- 2 cups cauliflower rice
- 2 teaspoons sesame oil
- Sea salt and freshly ground black pepper, to your liking
- 2 eggs, beaten
- 2 scallions, white and green parts separated, chopped
- 1 tablespoon Shoyu sauce
- 1 tablespoon sake
- 2 tablespoons Kewpie Japanese mayonnaise

Directions:
1. Thoroughly combine the cauliflower rice, sesame oil, salt, and pepper in a baking dish.
2. Cook at 340 degrees F about 13 minutes, stirring halfway through the cooking time.
3. Pour the eggs over the cauliflower rice and continue to cook about 5 minutes. Next, add the scallions and stir to combine. Continue to cook 2 to 3 minutes longer or until everything is heated through.
4. Meanwhile, make the sauce by whisking the Shoyu sauce, sake, and Japanese mayonnaise in a mixing bowl.
5. Divide the fried cauliflower rice between individual bowls and serve with the prepared sauce. Enjoy!

578.Baked Eggs With Cheese And Cauli Rice

Servings: 4
Cooking Time: 30 Minutes
Ingredients:
- 1 pound cauliflower rice

- 1 onion, diced
- 6 slices bacon, precooked
- 1 tablespoon butter, melted
- Sea salt and ground black pepper, to taste
- 6 eggs
- 1 cup cheddar cheese, shredded

Directions:
1. Place the cauliflower rice and onion in a lightly greased casserole dish. Add the bacon and the reserved quinoa. Drizzle the melted butter over cauliflower rice and sprinkle with salt and pepper.
2. Bake in the preheated Air Fryer at 390 degrees F for 10 minutes.
3. Turn the temperature down to 350 degrees F.
4. Make six indents for the eggs; crack one egg into each indent. Bake for 10 minutes, rotating the pan once or twice to ensure even cooking.
5. Top with cheese and bake for a further 5 minutes. Enjoy!

579.Parmesan Broccoli Fritters

Servings: 6
Cooking Time: 30 Minutes
Ingredients:
- 1 1/2 cups Monterey Jack cheese
- 1 teaspoon dried dill weed
- 1/3 teaspoon ground black pepper
- 3 eggs, whisked
- 1 teaspoon cayenne pepper
- 1/2 teaspoon kosher salt
- 2 ½ cups broccoli florets
- 1/2 cup Parmesan cheese

Directions:
1. Blitz the broccoli florets in a food processor until finely crumbed. Then, combine the broccoli with the rest of the above ingredients.
2. Roll the mixture into small balls; place the balls in the fridge for approximately half an hour.
3. Preheat your Air Fryer to 335 degrees F and set the timer to 14 minutes; cook until broccoli croquettes are browned and serve warm.

580.Country-style Apple Fries

Servings: 4
Cooking Time: 20 Minutes
Ingredients:
- 1/2 cup milk
- 1 egg
- 1/2 all-purpose flour
- 1 teaspoon baking powder
- 4 tablespoons brown sugar
- 1 teaspoon vanilla extract
- 1/2 teaspoon ground cloves

- A pinch of kosher salt
- A pinch of grated nutmeg
- 1 tablespoon coconut oil, melted
- 2 Pink Lady apples, cored, peeled, slice into pieces (shape and size of French fries
- 1/3 cup granulated sugar
- 1 teaspoon ground cinnamon

Directions:
1. In a mixing bowl, whisk the milk and eggs; gradually stir in the flour; add the baking powder, brown sugar, vanilla, cloves, salt, nutmeg, and melted coconut oil. Mix to combine well.
2. Dip each apple slice into the batter, coating on all sides. Spritz the bottom of the cooking basket with cooking oil.
3. Cook the apple fries in the preheated Air Fryer at 395 degrees F approximately 8 minutes, turning them over halfway through the cooking time.
4. Cook in small batches to ensure even cooking.
5. In the meantime, mix the granulated sugar with the ground cinnamon; sprinkle the cinnamon sugar over the apple fries. Serve warm.

581.Spicy Peppery Egg Salad

Servings: 3
Cooking Time: 20 Minutes + Chilling Time
Ingredients:
- 6 eggs
- 1 teaspoon mustard
- 1/2 cup mayonnaise
- 1 tablespoon white vinegar
- 1 habanero pepper, minced
- 1 red bell pepper, seeded and sliced
- 1 green bell pepper, seeded and sliced
- 1 shallot, sliced
- Sea salt and ground black pepper, to taste

Directions:
1. Place the wire rack in the Air Fryer basket; lower the eggs onto the wire rack.
2. Cook at 270 degrees F for 15 minutes.
3. Transfer them to an ice-cold water bath to stop the cooking. Peel the eggs under cold running water; coarsely chop the hard-boiled eggs and set aside.
4. Toss with the remaining ingredients and serve well chilled. Bon appétit!

582.Easy Frittata With Mozzarella And Kale

Servings: 3
Cooking Time: 20 Minutes
Ingredients:
- 1 yellow onion, finely chopped
- 6 ounces wild mushrooms, sliced
- 6 eggs

- 1/4 cup double cream
- 1/2 teaspoon cayenne pepper
- Sea salt and ground black pepper, to taste
- 1 tablespoon butter, melted
- 2 tablespoons fresh Italian parsley, chopped
- 2 cups kale, chopped
- 1/2 cup mozzarella, shredded

Directions:
1. Begin by preheating the Air Fryer to 360 degrees F. Spritz the sides and bottom of a baking pan with cooking oil.
2. Add the onions and wild mushrooms, and cook in the preheated Air Fryer at 360 degrees F for 4 to 5 minutes.
3. In a mixing dish, whisk the eggs and double cream until pale. Add the spices, butter, parsley, and kale; stir until everything is well incorporated.
4. Pour the mixture into the baking pan with the mushrooms.
5. Top with the cheese. Cook in the preheated Air Fryer for 10 minutes. Serve immediately and enjoy!

583.Frittata With Porcini Mushrooms

Servings: 4
Cooking Time: 40 Minutes
Ingredients:
- 3 cups Porcini mushrooms, thinly sliced
- 1 tablespoon melted butter
- 1 shallot, peeled and slice into thin rounds
- 1 garlic cloves, peeled and finely minced
- 1 lemon grass, cut into 1-inch pieces
- 1/3 teaspoon table salt
- 8 eggs
- 1/2 teaspoon ground black pepper, preferably freshly ground
- 1 teaspoon cumin powder
- 1/3 teaspoon dried or fresh dill weed
- 1/2 cup goat cheese, crumbled

Directions:
1. Melt the butter in a nonstick skillet that is placed over medium heat. Sauté the shallot, garlic, thinly sliced Porcini mushrooms, and lemon grass over a moderate heat until they have softened. Now, reserve the sautéed mixture.
2. Preheat your Air Fryer to 335 degrees F. Then, in a mixing bowl, beat the eggs until frothy. Now, add the seasonings and mix to combine well.
3. Coat the sides and bottom of a baking dish with a thin layer of vegetable spray. Pour the egg/seasoning mixture into the baking dish; throw in the onion/mushroom sauté. Top with the crumbled goat cheese.
4. Place the baking dish in the Air Fryer cooking basket. Cook for about 32 minutes or until your frittata is set. Enjoy!

584.Super-easy Chicken With Tomato Sauce

Servings: 4
Cooking Time: 20 Minutes + Marinating Time
Ingredients:
- 1 tablespoon balsamic vinegar
- ½ teaspoon red pepper flakes, crushed
- 1 fresh garlic, roughly chopped
- 2 ½ large-sized chicken breasts, cut into halves
- 1/3 handful fresh cilantro, roughly chopped
- 2 tablespoons olive oil
- 4 Roma tomatoes, diced
- 1 ½ tablespoons butter
- 1/3 handful fresh basil, loosely packed, sniped
- 1 teaspoon kosher salt
- 2 cloves garlic, minced
- Cooked bucatini, to serve

Directions:
1. Place the first seven ingredients in a medium-sized bowl; let it marinate for a couple of hours.
2. Preheat the air fryer to 325 degrees F. Air-fry your chicken for 32 minutes and serve warm.
3. In the meantime, prepare the tomato sauce by preheating a deep saucepan. Simmer the tomatoes until you make a chunky mixture. Throw in the garlic, basil, and butter; give it a good stir.
4. Serve the cooked chicken breasts with the tomato sauce and the cooked bucatini. Bon appétit!

585.Carrot Fries With Romano Cheese

Servings: 3
Cooking Time: 20 Minutes
Ingredients:
- 3 carrots, sliced into sticks
- 1 tablespoon coconut oil
- 1/3 cup Romano cheese, preferably freshly grated
- 2 teaspoons granulated garlic
- Sea salt and ground black pepper, to taste

Directions:
1. Toss all ingredients in a mixing bowl until the carrots are coated on all sides.
2. Cook at 380 degrees F for 15 minutes, shaking the basket halfway through the cooking time.
3. Serve with your favorite dipping sauce. Bon appétit!

586.Eggs With Turkey Bacon And Green Onions

Servings: 4
Cooking Time: 25 Minutes

Ingredients:
- 1/2 pound turkey bacon
- 4 eggs
- 1/3 cup milk
- 2 tablespoons yogurt
- 1/2 teaspoon sea salt
- 1 bell pepper, finely chopped
- 2 green onions, finely chopped
- 1/2 cup Colby cheese, shredded

Directions:
1. Place the turkey bacon in the cooking basket.
2. Cook at 360 degrees F for 9 to 11 minutes. Work in batches. Reserve the fried bacon.
3. In a mixing bowl, thoroughly whisk the eggs with milk and yogurt. Add salt, bell pepper, and green onions.
4. Brush the sides and bottom of the baking pan with the reserved 1 teaspoon of bacon grease.
5. Pour the egg mixture into the baking pan. Cook at 355 degrees F about 5 minutes. Top with shredded Colby cheese and cook for 5 to 6 minutes more.
6. Serve the scrambled eggs with the reserved bacon and enjoy!

587.Cheese And Chive Stuffed Chicken Rolls

Servings: 6
Cooking Time: 20 Minutes
Ingredients:
- 2 eggs, well-whisked
- Tortilla chips, crushed
- 1 1/2 tablespoons extra-virgin olive oil
- 1 ½ tablespoons fresh chives, chopped
- 3 chicken breasts, halved lengthwise
- 1 ½ cup soft cheese
- 2 teaspoons sweet paprika
- 1/2 teaspoon whole grain mustard
- 1/2 teaspoon cumin powder
- 1/3 teaspoon fine sea salt
- 1/3 cup fresh cilantro, chopped
- 1/3 teaspoon freshly ground black pepper, or more to taste

Directions:
1. Flatten out each piece of the chicken breast using a rolling pin. Then, grab three mixing dishes.
2. In the first one, combine the soft cheese with the cilantro, fresh chives, cumin, and mustard.
3. In another mixing dish, whisk the eggs together with the sweet paprika. In the third dish, combine the salt, black pepper, and crushed tortilla chips.
4. Spread the cheese mixture over each piece of chicken. Repeat with the remaining pieces of the chicken breasts; now, roll them up.
5. Coat each chicken roll with the whisked egg; dredge each chicken roll into the tortilla chips mixture. Lower the rolls onto the air fryer cooking basket. Drizzle extra-virgin olive oil over all rolls.
6. Air fry at 345 degrees F for 28 minutes, working in batches. Serve warm, garnished with sour cream if desired.

588.Red Currant Cupcakes

Servings: 3
Cooking Time: 20 Minutes
Ingredients:
- 1 cup all-purpose flour
- 1/2 cup sugar
- 1 teaspoon baking powder
- A pinch of kosher salt
- A pinch of grated nutmeg
- 1/4 cup coconut, oil melted
- 1 egg
- 1/4 cup full-fat coconut milk
- 1/4 teaspoon ground cardamom
- 1/4 teaspoon ground cinnamon
- 1 teaspoon vanilla extract
- 6 ounces red currants

Directions:
1. Mix the flour with the sugar, baking powder, salt, and nutmeg. In a separate bowl, whisk the coconut oil, egg, milk, cardamom, cinnamon, and vanilla.
2. Add the egg mixture to the dry ingredients; mix to combine well.
3. Now, fold in the red currants; gently stir to combine. Scrape the batter into lightly greased 6 standard-size muffin cups.
4. Bake your cupcakes at 360 degrees F for 12 minutes or until the tops are golden brown. Sprinkle some extra icing sugar over the top of each muffin if desired. Enjoy!

589.Masala-style Baked Eggs

Servings: 6
Cooking Time: 25 Minutes
Ingredients:
- 6 medium-sized eggs, beaten
- 1 teaspoon garam masala
- 1 cup scallions, finely chopped
- 3 cloves garlic, finely minced
- 2 cups leftover chicken, shredded
- 2 tablespoons sesame oil
- Hot sauce, for drizzling
- 1 teaspoon turmeric
- 1 teaspoon mixed peppercorns, freshly cracked
- 1 teaspoon kosher salt
- 1/3 teaspoon smoked paprika

Directions:

1. Warm sesame oil in a sauté pan over a moderate flame; then, sauté the scallions together with garlic until just fragrant; it takes about 5 minutes. Now, throw in leftover chicken and stir until thoroughly warmed.
2. In a medium-sized bowl or a measuring cup, thoroughly combine the eggs with all seasonings.
3. Then, coat the inside of six oven safe ramekins with a nonstick cooking spray. Divide the egg/chicken mixture among your ramekins.
4. Air-fry approximately 18 minutes at 355 degrees F. Drizzle with hot sauce and eat warm.

590.Celery And Bacon Cakes

Servings: 4
Cooking Time: 25 Minutes
Ingredients:
- 2 eggs, lightly beaten
- 1/3 teaspoon freshly cracked black pepper
- 1 cup Colby cheese, grated
- 1/2 tablespoon fresh dill, finely chopped
- 1/2 tablespoon garlic paste
- 1/3 cup onion, finely chopped
- 1/3 cup bacon, chopped
- 2 teaspoons fine sea salt
- 2 medium-sized celery stalks, trimmed and grated
- 1/3 teaspoon baking powder

Directions:
1. Place the celery on a paper towel and squeeze them to remove the excess liquid.
2. Combine the vegetables with the other ingredients in the order listed above. Shape the balls using 1 tablespoon of the vegetable mixture.
3. Then, gently flatten each ball with your palm or a wide spatula. Spritz the croquettes with a nonstick cooking oil.
4. Bake the vegetable cakes in a single layer for 17 minutes at 318 degrees F. Serve warm with sour cream.

591.Dinner Turkey Sandwiches

Servings: 4
Cooking Time: 4 Hours 30 Minutes
Ingredients:
- 1/2 pound turkey breast
- 1 teaspoon garlic powder
- 7 ounces condensed cream of onion soup
- 1/3 teaspoon ground allspice
- BBQ sauce, to savor

Directions:
1. Simply dump the cream of onion soup and turkey breast into your crock-pot. Cook on HIGH heat setting for 3 hours.

2. Then, shred the meat and transfer to a lightly greased baking dish.
3. Pour in your favorite BBQ sauce. Sprinkle with ground allspice and garlic powder. Air-fry an additional 28 minutes.
4. To finish, assemble the sandwiches; add toppings such as pickled or fresh salad, mustard, etc.

592.Easy Cheesy Broccoli

Servings: 4
Cooking Time: 25 Minutes
Ingredients:
- 1/3 cup grated yellow cheese
- 1 large-sized head broccoli, stemmed and cut small florets
- 2 1/2 tablespoons canola oil
- 2 teaspoons dried rosemary
- 2 teaspoons dried basil
- Salt and ground black pepper, to taste

Directions:
1. Bring a medium pan filled with a lightly salted water to a boil. Then, boil the broccoli florets for about 3 minutes.
2. Then, drain the broccoli florets well; toss them with the canola oil, rosemary, basil, salt and black pepper.
3. Set your air fryer to 390 degrees F; arrange the seasoned broccoli in the cooking basket; set the timer for 17 minutes. Toss the broccoli halfway through the cooking process.
4. Serve warm topped with grated cheese and enjoy!

593.Cajun Turkey Meatloaf

Servings: 6
Cooking Time: 45 Minutes
Ingredients:
- 1 1/3 pounds turkey breasts, ground
- ½ cup vegetable stock
- 2 eggs, lightly beaten
- 1/2 sprig thyme, chopped
- 1/2 teaspoon Cajun seasonings
- 1/2 sprig coriander, chopped
- ½ cup seasoned breadcrumbs
- 2 tablespoons butter, room temperature
- 1/2 cup scallions, chopped
- 1/3 teaspoon ground nutmeg
- 1/3 cup tomato ketchup
- 1/2 teaspoon table salt
- 2 teaspoons whole grain mustard
- 1/3 teaspoon mixed peppercorns, freshly cracked

Directions:
1. Firstly, warm the butter in a medium-sized saucepan that is placed over a moderate heat; sauté the scallions together with the

chopped thyme and coriander leaves until just tender.
2. While the scallions are sautéing, set your air fryer to cook at 365 degrees F.
3. Combine all the ingredients, minus the ketchup, in a mixing dish; fold in the sautéed mixture and mix again.
4. Shape into a meatloaf and top with the tomato ketchup. Air-fry for 50 minutes. Bon appétit!

594.Mozzarella Stick Nachos

Servings: 4
Cooking Time: 40 Minutes
Ingredients:
- 1 (16-ounce) package mozzarella cheese sticks
- 2 eggs
- 1/2 cup flour
- 1/2 (7 12-ounce bag multigrain tortilla chips, crushed
- 1 teaspoon garlic powder
- 1 teaspoon dried oregano
- 1/2 cup salsa, preferably homemade
-

Directions:
1. Set up your breading station. Put the flour into a shallow bowl; beat the eggs in another shallow bowl; in a third bowl, mix the crushed tortilla chips, garlic powder, and oregano.
2. Coat the mozzarella sticks lightly with flour, followed by the egg, and then the tortilla chips mixture. Place in your freezer for 30 minutes.
3. Place the breaded cheese sticks in the lightly greased Air Fryer basket. Cook at 380 degrees F for 6 minutes.
4. Serve with salsa on the side and enjoy!

595.Gruyère Stuffed Mushrooms

Servings: 3
Cooking Time: 19 Minutes
Ingredients:
- 2 garlic cloves, minced
- 1 teaspoon ground black pepper, or more to taste
- 1/2 teaspoon paprika
- 1 teaspoon dried parsley flakes
- 1½ tablespoons fresh mint, chopped
- 1 teaspoon salt, or more to taste
- 1 cup Gruyère cheese, shredded
- 9 large mushrooms, cleaned, stalks removed

Directions:
1. Mix all of the above ingredients, minus the mushrooms, in a mixing bowl to prepare the filling.

2. Then, stuff the mushrooms with the prepared filling.
3. Air-fry stuffed mushrooms at 375 degrees F for about 12 minutes. Taste for doneness and serve at room temperature as an appetizer.

596.Spicy Potato Wedges

Servings: 4
Cooking Time: 23 Minutes
Ingredients:
- 1 ½ tablespoons melted butter
- 1 teaspoon dried parsley flakes
- 1 teaspoon ground coriander
- 1 teaspoon seasoned salt
- 3 large-sized red potatoes, cut into wedges
- 1/2 teaspoon chili powder
- 1/3 teaspoon garlic pepper

Directions:
1. Dump the potato wedges into the air fryer cooking basket. Drizzle with melted butter and cook for 20 minutes at 380 degrees F. Make sure to shake them a couple of times during the cooking process.
2. Add the remaining ingredients; toss to coat potato wedges on all sides. Bon appétit!

597.Potato And Kale Croquettes

Servings: 6
Cooking Time: 9 Minutes
Ingredients:
- 4 eggs, slightly beaten
- 1/3 cup flour
- 1/3 cup goat cheese, crumbled
- 1 ½ teaspoons fine sea salt
- 4 garlic cloves, minced
- 1 cup kale, steamed
- 1/3 cup breadcrumbs
- 1/3teaspoon red pepper flakes
- 3 potatoes, peeled and quartered
- 1/3 teaspoon dried dill weed

Directions:
1. Firstly, boil the potatoes in salted water. Once the potatoes are cooked, mash them; add the kale, goat cheese, minced garlic, sea salt, red pepper flakes, dill and one egg; stir to combine well.
2. Now, roll the mixture to form small croquettes.
3. Grab three shallow bowls. Place the flour in the first shallow bowl.
4. Beat the remaining 3 eggs in the second bowl. After that, throw the breadcrumbs into the third shallow bowl.
5. Dip each croquette in the flour; then, dip them in the eggs bowl; lastly, roll each croquette in the breadcrumbs.

6. Air fry at 335 degrees F for 7 minutes or until golden. Tate, adjust for seasonings and serve warm.

598.Italian Eggs With Smoked Salmon

Servings: 4
Cooking Time: 25 Minutes
Ingredients:
- 1/3 cup Asiago cheese, grated
- 1/3 teaspoon dried dill weed
- 1/2 tomato, chopped
- 6 eggs
- 1/3 cup milk
- Pan spray
- 1 cup smoked salmon, chopped
- Fine sea salt and freshly cracked black pepper, to taste
- 1/3 teaspoon smoked cayenne pepper

Directions:
1. Set your air fryer to cook at 365 degrees F. In a mixing bowl, whisk the eggs, milk, smoked cayenne pepper, salt, black pepper, and dill weed.
2. Lightly grease 4 ramekins with pan spray of choice; divide the egg/milk mixture among the prepared ramekins.
3. Add the salmon and tomato; top with the grated Asiago cheese. Finally, air-fry for 16 minutes. Bon appétit!

599.Veggie Casserole With Ham And Baked Eggs

Servings: 4
Cooking Time: 30 Minutes
Ingredients:
- 2 tablespoons butter, melted
- 1 zucchini, diced
- 1 bell pepper, seeded and sliced
- 1 red chili pepper, seeded and minced
- 1 medium-sized leek, sliced
- 3/4 pound ham, cooked and diced
- 5 eggs
- 1 teaspoon cayenne pepper
- Sea salt, to taste
- 1/2 teaspoon ground black pepper
- 1 tablespoon fresh cilantro, chopped

Directions:
1. Start by preheating the Air Fryer to 380 degrees F. Grease the sides and bottom of a baking pan with the melted butter.
2. Place the zucchini, peppers, leeks and ham in the baking pan. Bake in the preheated Air Fryer for 6 minutes.
3. Crack the eggs on top of ham and vegetables; season with the cayenne pepper, salt, and black pepper. Bake for a further 20 minutes or until the whites are completely set.
4. Garnish with fresh cilantro and serve. Bon appétit!

600.Peanut Butter And Chicken Bites

Servings: 8
Cooking Time: 10 Minutes
Ingredients:
- 1 ½ tablespoons soy sauce
- 1/2 teaspoon smoked cayenne pepper
- 8 ounces soft cheese
- 1 1/2 tablespoons peanut butter
- 1/3 leftover chicken
- 1 teaspoon sea salt
- 32 wonton wrappers
- 1/3 teaspoon freshly cracked mixed peppercorns
- 1/2 tablespoon pear cider vinegar

Directions:
1. Combine all of the above ingredients, minus the wonton wrappers, in a mixing dish.
2. Lay out the wrappers on a clean surface. Now, spread the wonton wrappers with the prepared chicken filling.
3. Fold the outside corners to the center over the filling; after that, roll up the wrappers tightly; you can moisten the edges with a little water.
4. Set the air fryer to cook at 360 degrees F. Air fry the rolls for 6 minutes, working in batches. Serve with marinara sauce. Bon appétit!

Milton Keynes UK
Ingram Content Group UK Ltd.
UKHW050010191223
434628UK00007B/437

9 781922 547590